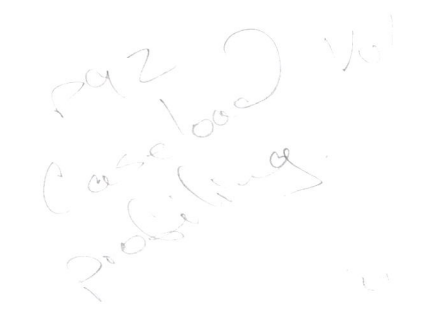

Skill Mix in Health Visiting and Community Nursing Teams
Principles into Practice

Maggie Fisher

The author

Maggie has worked as a health visitor for twenty seven years both in London and Hampshire. She is co-chair of the Unite/CPHVA Special Interest and Development Group for Parenting and Family Support and chair of the Unite/CPHVA Health Visitor Forum. Maggie was seconded to work part time as a Professional Officer at Unite/CPHVA from April 2007-December 2008 during which time she prepared this book on Skill Mix in Health Visiting and Community Nursing Teams. She has recently taken up a new post funded by the Department for Children, Schools and Families working as a health visitor with Netmums as part of their Parent Know How Project

Maggie Fisher. RGN. NDN. RHV. BA (Hons) Ed. PG Diploma.
Lead Local Coordinator, Netmums and Chair of Unite/CPHVA Health Visitors' Forum.

Published by:
Unite the Union/The Community Practitioners' and Health Visitors' Association
The Health Sector
Unite the Union
124 Theobalds Rd
London, WC1X 8TN
Telephone: 020 7611 2500

www,.unitetheunion.org/cphva
www.cphvabookshop.com

The Community Practitioners' and Health Visitors' Association (CPHVA) is a professional section of Unite Health Sector which has about 100,000 members working in the health sector. Unite/CPHVA is the third largest professional nursing union and is the only union which has public health at its heart. Unite/CPHVA is the UK professional body that represents registered nurses, nursery nurses and health visitors who work in a primary or community health setting.

The sector is itself part of the Unite trade union with 2 million members nationwide. Unite the Union was formed by an amalgamation of Amicus and the Transport and General Workers' Union in May 2007.

© Unite the Union. No part of this publication may be reproduced, stored in a retrieval system or transmitted by electronic or other means without the consent of Unite the Union. All rights reserved.

October 2009

ISBN: 1-872278-75-2

Contents

vi   Foreword

1   Introduction

3   **Chapter 1: Understanding the concept of skill mix**
Context
Policy drivers
What is skill mix?
Rationale for introducing skill mix
Evidence base for skill mix

26   **Chapter 2: Integrated children's services**
Improving skills and standards within integrated children's services
The Integrated Qualifications Framework (IQF)
National Occupational Standards for Working with Parents
Common Core of Skills and Knowledge for the Children's Workforce
Standards for Better Health

34   **Chapter 3: The realities of skill mix in the workplace: issues for professionals in practice**
Professional regulation
Accountability
Delegation
Information sharing
Confidentiality
Informed client consent

60   **Chapter 4: Introducing skill mix – considerations for practise**
Models
Considerations for practice
Safeguarding children – a public health priority
The population paradox

70   **Conclusion**

72   **Recommendations**

74   **Frequently asked questions**

93   References

102   Relevant CPHVA publications for additional reading

103   Glossary

Foreword

No-one can argue against the fact that resources in the public sector are finite. Therefore, it is essential to challenge the evidence base for the way services are designed and delivered. In all my years in professional practice and my 10 years working for Unite the Union and the Community Practitioners' & Health Visitors' Association, no single topic has caused as much professional debate as the introduction of skill mix into health visiting and community nursing. It was marketed to professionals as a method for ensuring that high level professional skills could be targeted to where they would be most effective. Furthermore, that time would be freed up to develop additional services for the public. Unfortunately our members tell us that in many instances the opposite is the case. Skill mix has been used as a method of "balancing the books" and any assessment of its impact on the quality of services has rarely featured in decision making. Of more concern, issues regarding accountability in relation to delegation have not been taken seriously, leaving many of our members very anxious about the high levels of responsibility imposed on them.

At the end of the day the beneficiaries of NHS services are the public. It is they and their families who will feel the impact of inappropriate skill mix. In the case of public health practice, the repercussions may be long term and even affect future generations. Managers have to balance the books in the short term but this book makes clear the potential financial impact for the NHS and society in the longer term in getting it wrong. Unite/CPHVA supports the use of proper skill mix but not grade mix or skill substitution, where the team is left with insufficient senior or advanced skills.

We welcome this excellent book written by Maggie Fisher when she was a valued part of the Unite Health Sector professional team, and informed by members of our Health Visiting Forum. We believe that it will provide our members and others with the information to ensure the right balance of professional and other skills either in teams they are part of, or responsible for.

Whilst the book particularly focuses on health visiting where most concerns have been raised by our members, much of the content is just as relevant for school and district nursing and other community health teams.

Dr Cheryll Adams
Lead Professional Officer, Strategy and Practice Development, 2009

Introduction

Skill mix has been the subject of much debate in community nursing since the early '90s when a report into skill mix in district nursing by the Value for Money Unit (VFM) was published (NHS Executive, 1992). At the time Cowley (1993) warned of the dangers inherent in this "simplistic value for money approach to skill mix in community nursing teams". The VFM (NHS Executive, 1992) attempted to reduce elements of primary care to a series of mechanised tasks that could be counted and reallocated. Contacts were measured in terms of activity rather than in terms of health outcomes or best value. In the VFM model, skilled district nurses were expected to delegate the core of their work to relatively unskilled workers, reducing their clinical input to more of a supervisory or managerial role. There is significant concern that the narrowing of experience of the senior professionals runs the risk of deskilling them, reducing their clinical ability, and putting patients at risk, in addition to lowering morale (McKenna, 1998). For example, if practitioners lose their generic role and spend the majority of their time on supervision and staff management, or only visiting more complex clients or families, they will lose their generic skills and become deskilled in this area.

The rationale for introducing skill mix is to allocate skills to those practitioners capable of undertaking them effectively at the least cost to the service and reduce the need for skilled clinical practitioners to do activities which another member of staff is better skilled to do, for example administrative and clerical duties. There is also substantial evidence that a rich skill mix of mostly qualified staff is a highly effective and efficient way to run a health service (McKenna, 1995). Health visiting teams are no longer expected to work in homogenous groups but rather work in integrated teams with other health and local authority workers to provide an integrated service to children and families. This leaves the profession with no option but to embrace new skill mix practices. What is important however, is that they are involved in determining the most effective skill mix formula to provide safe quality care to their clients.

A professional briefing *Delegation and Professional Accountability* (CPHVA, 2002) addressed some of the issues raised by the introduction of skill mix in health visiting. Since then Unite/CPHVA has been inundated with calls for further guidance as cash-strapped PCTs and employing authorities have sought to increase the use of skill mix and have introduced grade mix in health visiting and primary health care teams in an apparent attempt to cut costs. The Nursing & Midwifery Council (NMC) has also reported a sharp increase in the number of enquiries relating to delegation, specifically with regards to non-regulated health care staff (NMC Press Release, 2007).

The cost of staffing the NHS amounts to 70% of NHS spending and many managers are under pressure to reduce costs. The attractions of reducing staffing costs by delegating tasks to the lowest grades who can perform such functions are obvious. Not surprisingly health professionals in district nursing, midwifery, school nursing, health

Introduction

visiting and other allied professions in health and social care have expressed concern over what they view is the subsequent gradual erosion of the quality of care.

Skill mix, if used appropriately can free practitioners' time for professional and practitioner role development and result in increased job satisfaction and improvements in the work/life balance.

Team working can make a substantial contribution to improvements in patient care and align services more effectively and appropriately to the health needs of the local population.

Skill mix can also be an efficient use of scarce resources and help to compensate for the reduced number of skilled professionals in the community e.g. the reduction in the numbers of health visitors who have been trained and the older age profile of the workforce. However, for skill mix to be acceptable there needs to be evidence that it is cost effective, safe and satisfactory to both users and practitioners. It is important to consider these criteria together as a variation in one may have implications for the others. The lack of robust evidence for a safe and effective skill mix formula is one of the main professional concerns regarding its use. It is important that services should be predicated on evidence and not just solely economic considerations.

There are many excellent examples of successful skill mix teams in community health care across the country. These illustrate how community practitioners can capitalise on the potential of skill mix to enhance service provision for children and families.

It is hoped that this book will be a useful practical guide for any staff involved in skill mix working, development or implementation. It aims to explore many of the issues which Unite/CPHVA members have requested information on over the last few years in relation to skill mix.

Acknowledgements

Very many people become involved in producing a book such as this and it is impossible to personally thank them all. I would particularly like to make reference though to my colleagues on the Unite/CPHVA Health Visitor Forum who were very influential in the early stages as the content was decided and in peer reviewing the early drafts. Thanks must also be given to Cheryll Adams, Lead Professional Officer, who worked tirelessly to get the book to press after my secondment to the CPHVA came to an end. Finally I must thank my family for their forbearance when I frequently worked into the night and at weekends to complete it.

Maggie Fisher, *October 2009*

1 Understanding the concept of skill mix

This chapter defines skill mix and explores the contextual and policy background to skill mix and the rational behind its introduction. It also examines the evidence base for skill mix and the advantages and professional concerns associated with its introduction into community practice.

Context

In recent years there has been an enormous growth in professional knowledge and technical advances in all areas of nursing and public health practice. Cowley and Frost (2006) identified that there is now more specialist knowledge within each role and, paradoxically, there is also more in common across health care roles than ever before (Warner, Gould and Picek 1998).

To ensure that specialist professional knowledge is shared will necessitate an increase in inter-professional teamwork with different team members holding a common core of knowledge and each making a specific contribution to the overall task of the team and care of patients/clients and families.

Although skill mix is still somewhat in its infancy in health visiting practice, it has been around a long time in "clinical" nurse practice in the hospital setting and in other more clinical type roles in the community. It is necessary, therefore, to explore which have been the major drivers that have influenced its introduction into health visiting and, furthermore, attempt to make sense of what we understand by skill mix in this context.

Policy drivers

The evolving nature of health care in the United Kingdom has been influenced by a number of factors including; demographics – both of patients and the workforce looking after them, finite resources and new technologies. All of these have impacted on government policy, which influences the way health care is delivered in the community.

In response to ongoing changes the Nursing & Midwifery Council (NMC) and Department of Health (DH) have recently reviewed the future of pre and post registration nursing education respectively in the UK. This was to ensure the future nursing workforce will be prepared to meet the challenges of providing health care in the next two decades and beyond. The recommendations from these reviews will undoubtedly have impact on the evolution of skill mix in the future.

Understanding the concept of skill mix

The changing population demographics, increased life expectancy and dependency ratios all indicate that a radical rethink of the way health care professionals are trained and deployed is needed. We are likely to see an expansion of telecare to support care at home, with new applications of biotechnology, bioengineering and robotics (Longley *et al*, 2007). Care will be focussed in the community with an increasing emphasis on the provision of care closer to home and self-care to support the increasing number of people with long-term conditions. *Modernising Nursing Careers* (DH, 2006) a review of how nursing needs to be modernised across the 4 countries of the UK to meet current and evolving health needs, suggested that nursing in primary care environments will be a greater focus of future nursing career pathways with a greater emphasis on prevention, health promotion and self-care.

Government health policy across the UK recognises the need to devolve care away from hospitals and in to the local community. Developing medical technology and the progression towards shorter hospital stays, day surgery, the management of complex conditions and the care of children who have life-limiting/threatening illnesses requiring to be managed in the home environment, has led to an increased demand for 24-hour care in the community. Financial imperatives have a crucial influence on the shape of any health care system and there is an increased emphasis on giving patients/clients choice in where they access health care.

This shift away from hospital-based care requires an increase in the range and mix of skills in primary health care teams (PHCTs) to meet these demands. There is a blurring of professional boundaries reflected both in policy documents and in practice, with an emphasis on the need to make the best use of scarce resources.

Promoting public health and children's well-being is no longer solely the domain of the NHS or Children's Services departments. Many other statutory, community and voluntary agencies are now central to this agenda. School and education play an integral part in community development as highlighted by the expansion of extended schools and Children's Centres in local communities, which will provide integrated health and social care. This emphasis in multi-agency working and the pooling of budgets has encouraged the development of new ways of working together. This is resulting in different configurations in the make-up of skill mix teams in the community, across the UK.

One of the challenges the NHS in England faces is how to integrate health and social care and personalise care for patients, children and families where possible. Health and social care is developing in different ways in the devolved countries. Northern Ireland has, for many years, successfully integrated services into the Department of Health, Social Services and Public Safety

Policy documents across the UK relating to families, children and community services emphasise the provision of services designed to suit the needs of families and young people receiving them rather than the professionals delivering them.

Skill mix working and teams of the future will need to ensure they fulfil this brief and provide services that are integrated and easy for families, children and young people to access and use. There is a requirement for all agencies working with children, young people and their families to work together to provide better outcomes for children and families.

Central to public health policy has been the focus on the importance of prevention and early interventions, fuelled by concerns over the rising costs of health care (Wanless, 2004) and health inequalities (DH, 2003, DH, 2004a). These and other policies represent a central theme of government strategy to support mothers, fathers, families and children, which was reflected in the review of the role of health visitors in England (DH, 2007). Supporting mothers and fathers to attuned parenting in particular during the first months of life, has also been a major theme across UK government policy.

The *NHS Constitution* (DH, 2009) establishes the principles and values of the NHS in England and sets out commitments to patients, public and staff in the form of rights to which they are entitled, and pledges which the NHS will strive to deliver. The Government will be required by law to renew the NHS Constitution every 10 years, with the full involvement of the patients who use the health service, the public who fund it and the staff who work in it. All NHS organisations will be required to take account of the NHS Constitution in the decisions that they make.

From a community perspective, this NHS Constitution could be a very powerful lever for community practitioners and the communities they serve in the bid to ensure quality services. PCTs and employing authorities will be legally obliged to assess the health requirements of their communities and provide services to meet those needs. A similar ethos of commitment to high quality patient-focused care exists in the health policy agenda of the devolved countries of Northern Ireland, Wales and Scotland.

Employing authorities could potentially face a legal challenge brought by members of the public if they felt that they were not receiving an acceptable standard of care from their NHS provider. This could have serious implications for all involved in health and social care; in particular primary health care teams, health visiting, school nursing and maternity services. NHS providers will need to ensure that the skill mix they provide is acceptable to the public and users of the service.

Policy also focuses on personal and responsive health care – providing integrated care based around the person, not just their individual symptoms or care needs. Current strategy underlines the central role primary and community care services play in keeping people healthy, preventing illness and promoting healthy life styles as well as tackling regional variations in health and well-being. Further skill mix development and alternative models of providing care in the future will be heavily influenced by policy developments and evidence from practice.

KEY POINTS

1. Government policy will continue to influence the way skill mix is developed in the community.
2. The emphasis is on the provision of services designed to suit the needs of families and young people receiving them rather than the professionals delivering them. Skill mix teams of the future may have many workers from different backgrounds working together for example in Children's Centres and the Welsh Sure Start/Flying Start model. This will require new governance to ensure professionals from different

Understanding the concept of skill mix

agencies communicate effectively and all workers receive regular high quality supervision and ongoing professional development to safeguard the public.
3. If there are to be changes in the way that services are delivered that may affect continuity of care, then employing authorities are duty bound to involve and consult service users. All of the above provide powerful levers for community practitioners to use to advocate for safe, quality services for children and families that promote protect and improve their health. It is crucial that practitioners become familiar with the policy documents relating to their particular region/country and use them to safeguard quality services.

What is skill mix?

There are many different terms that have been used to describe skill mix including:

re-profiling, grade mix, substitution, collaboration, integrated teams and multi-skilling. Confusion often arises between the terms skill mix and grade mix (Cowley and Adams, 2009).

It is important to be clear about the term skill and our understanding of it.

Skill, as defined by the Concise Oxford Dictionary (Oxford University Press, 1978), has several meanings the one most appropriate to nursing and community practice is: *"Expertness, practised ability. Facility **in** an action, or **in** doing, or **to** do something"*.

Wikipedia provides the following definition:

> *"Skill is the learned capacity or talent to carry out pre-determined results often with the minimum outlay of time, energy, or both. Skills can often be divided into domain-general and domain-specific skills. For example, in the domain of work, some general skills would include **time management, teamwork,** and **leadership, self motivation** and others, whereas domain-specific skills would be useful only for a certain job. Skill often depends on numerous variables".*
> (Wikipedia, October 5th 2008)

The above two definitions emphasise the expertness, learnt capacity and practised ability in order to do something, or a cognitive ability to be able to function at a certain level of expertise in something that is domain specific. An example of this could be the general skills nurses acquire through their general nursing training, and the specific skills, knowledge and competencies acquired through post registration training that equip specialist community public health nurses to work in the community.

In nursing and Specialist Community Public Health Nursing (SCPHN), skill is associated with the knowledge, education and experience which equips an individual with a set of competencies which enables them to fulfil their role (Newland, 2009). The UKCC has previously used the term competency to describe *"...the **skills** and ability to practise safely and effectively without the need for direct supervision"*. (*Fitness for Practice*, UKCC, 1999)

The Code (NMC, 2008) states:

> "To practise competently, you must possess the knowledge, **skills** and abilities required for lawful, safe and effective practice without direct supervision. You must acknowledge the limits of your professional competence and only undertake practice and accept responsibilities for those activities in which you are competent".

Having considered the term skill, it is important to explore what is generally accepted to be the different features of grade mix and skill mix.

Gibbs *et al* (1991) defined grade mix as a mix of differing grades of staff in a particular working environment, their costs and activities. Grade mix does not reflect the skills of the staff concerned or the needs of their clients.

Skill mix refers to the skills and experience of staff, their continuing education and professional development, level of experience and how they bring these together to influence their professional judgement. Skill mix connects "needs" with skills available and outcomes in a particular working environment with a specific client group. The table below outlines the essential differences between grade and skill mix.

Table 1: The differences between skill mix and grade mix or skill substitution

Grade mix (skill substitution)	Skill mix
How much does the service cost?	What are the needs of the client group?
How can a different mix of grades do the same job more cheaply?	What mix of skill is needed to best address identified needs?
What parts of the work of more expensive grades can be done by cheaper grades?	Which groups of staff possess those skills?
	How can the team be organised to ensure appropriate allocation of responsibility?

Skill mix identifies what needs to be done and the skills required to do it. It involves identifying the professional who has the required skills and competencies to carry out the work. As can be seen from the above table, the purpose behind the introduction of grade or skill mix and how it is introduced and developed is of critical importance to its success or failure.

Skill mix can be a contentious issue and this has heightened the belief amongst some practitioners that managers do not always understand and value the complexity of the work and their knowledge and skill level (Morell, 1993). This is accentuated by a lack of available robust evidence into the cost effectiveness and safety of introducing skill mix. It is important for community practitioners, managers and commissioners of services to have a clear understanding of the essential differences between grade and skill mix and the implications this has for practice and the delivery of safe services.

Understanding the concept of skill mix

There have been no trials comparing the safety of working practices of different practitioners in skill mix teams compared to health visitors working in a traditional model, particularly in terms of safeguarding children, domestic abuse and the detection of postnatal depression.

As stated earlier, McKenna (1998) identified that the narrowing of experience of the senior professionals in skill mix teams runs the risk of deskilling them and reducing their clinical ability in addition to lowering morale.

These concerns highlight an urgent need for research to ascertain safe working practice in skill mix teams, and whether delegation of health visitor tasks to other health care team members affects the provision of "soft" areas of care such as health promotion or psychological support. There is evidence from general practice (Charlton *et al*, 1994) of significant unmet need especially with regard to aspects of health promotion and it is not clear whether skill mix teams are able to identify and meet these needs.

Carr and Pearson (2005) examined delegation in community nursing and explored some of the complex processes involved in making delegation decisions in skill mix. They also identified the potential reduction in the identification of need as a key issue in delegated decision making, which, when examined in detail, was extremely complex. In this study the research participants indicated that they would only delegate routine care, however this was problematic as it wasn't possible to differentiate what was routine and what was not. In a hospital setting the patient is captive in a controlled environment where staff of different grades may have input to the same patient during the course of a treatment. In the community an important factor in delegation decision making is the predictability of care, the response to risk and coping with uncertainty. In the home setting, only the delegate may be delivering care where there is a lack of opportunity to directly supervise care or advice given. The lack of a physical infrastructure that exists outside a hospital or GP practice setting causes extra delegation dilemmas for the community practitioner. Predictability of care is an important concept in health visiting and community nursing and is discussed in more detail in Chapter 3 which examines accountability and delegation.

The Health Visitors' Association (HVA now the CPHVA) identified that when skill mix was introduced through a "bottom-up" approach, with the full involvement of the health visiting or nursing team, and with a thorough review of the skills needed in a particular team, it could be very successful. Wright's (1998) study of skill mix identified that successful skill mix requires practitioner involvement. However, when grade mix is introduced to cut costs, provide solutions to recruitment difficulties, reduce the nursing budget and, is imposed by management on community teams, it is often unsuccessful.

KEY POINTS

1. Grade mix: a mix of differing grades of staff in a particular working environment, their costs and activities. Grade mix does not reflect the skills of the staff concerned or the needs of their clients (Gibbs *et al*, 1991).
2. Skill mix: the skills and experience of staff, their continuing education and professional development, years of experience and how they bring these together to influence their

professional judgement. Skill mix connects "needs" with skills available and outcomes, in a particular working environment, with a specific client group.
3. Skill mix and grade mix are very different; therefore it is important for community practitioners, managers and commissioners of services to have a clear understanding of the essential differences between the two and the implications this has for practice and the delivery of services.
4. Delegating work to relatively unskilled or junior workers runs the risk of deskilling senior staff, narrowing their experience and reducing their clinical ability in addition to lowering morale.

The differences between nursing and SCPHN: the implications for skill mix

One of the challenges that have fuelled the debate over skill mix is the vexed question of the differences between SCPHN and the nursing care of patients who have an illness or disability. It would seem, from the many enquires that Unite/CPHVA receive from members, that there is a degree of confusion over this from managers and commissioners of services who appear to assume that the skills of a staff nurse are interchangeable with those of a health visitor since all SCPHN have a nursing qualification as a prerequisite for obtaining a SCPHN qualification. Consequently, it is important that these essential differences are explored as it should help inform how skill mix staff may be used and deployed.

Getting the balance of skills right in the care setting which staff are working in is imperative if skill mix is to be used effectively and appropriately. There is evidence from practice to suggest that the SCPHN's preferred approach home visiting, community outreach and group support is very effective in reducing health inequalities (Unite/CPHVA response to the Marmot Review, 2009), this is a very different form of practice to general nursing and less open to skill mix. A recent Unite/CPHVA publication has demonstrated the scale of the differences (Newland, 2009).

All health visitors and qualified school nurses are both general nurses and SCPHNs; some may also be midwives. However, the main role and function of health visiting and school nursing is not clinical nursing in the traditional "medical model" of caring for the ill patient. It is concerned with the promotion of health and the prevention and early detection of disease. The majority of nurses provide care for people who are ill, dependent or disabled and often work closely with doctors who have overall responsibility for them. In contrast, health visitors and school nurses work with an undifferentiated caseload for which they have responsibility and accountability. Traditionally health visitors have set their own priorities and, in partnership with clients, decided their own visiting patterns using their professional judgement, rather than relying on medical direction.

Cowley and Cann (2007) conducted a survey of 1,456 health visitors to examine the work health visitors were actively engaged in. When asked how health visiting related to nursing, 57 % reported that it was completely different or somewhat different. When the respondents were asked how closely health visiting related to public health

Understanding the concept of skill mix

88 % said it was the same or somewhat similar. Cowley (2002) discusses many of the differences between nursing, health visiting and public health and identifies how different aspects of practice are operationalised within the different occupational groups. Health visiting and school nursing should not be regarded as a specialist part of nursing as they are essentially very different as these four aspects of practice identify:

1. Individual or collective focus; it is the individual or population needs that dominate the service provision.
2. The focus is on the determinants of health and health inequalities, or treating established problems.
3. The focus of care belong in the public and/or private domain.
4. It operates in a social or bio-medical model of health?

Health visitors and school nurses work both with individual children and families, and the local population; they are different from the majority of nurses as SCPHNs focus on well populations. Health visitors focus on the determinants of health and health inequalities at both an individual, local and general population level and will work to influence the policies which affect health at local, strategic and national level, indeed this is one of the *Principles of Health Visiting*. The search for health needs and the stimulation of the awareness of health needs (also *Principles of Health Visiting*) are done both in the private domain with individuals through home visiting, but also publicly through group work, health promotion and local and national campaigns.

SCPHN, whilst understanding the bio-medical model of health are much more focussed and interested in what creates health; they see health as a process that is ever-changing and dynamic; individuals at any one time may be heading towards well-being or illness. The role and function – and the fourth and underpinning principle of health visiting – is to facilitate health enhancing activities and enable the individual/family to maintain or recover their health equilibrium and progress towards achieving health and well-being. The different aspects of the principles of practice outlined above illustrate how fundamentally different a health visiting approach is to a nursing one and that SCPHNs do not simply do nursing in a public health way (Newland, 2009).

If skill mix staff are to be used in a cost effective and appropriate way it is vital that commissioners and managers of services have a clear understanding of SCPHNs' unique skills (Unite/CPHVA 2008; Newland 2009). The post-registration SCPHN training that practitioners undergo significantly equips them to radically alter their approach to working in public health practice and family well-being. The combination of family welfare and public health knowledge required to work with individuals, families and communities is unique and only provided by SCPHNs. It has a very different emphasis from that provided by a children's or adult nurse and requires a high level of professional skill. This is very important in relation to safeguarding vulnerable children and adults, the detection of postnatal depression, domestic abuse, and, in the search for and the identification of, need. The 2008 Netmums Survey (Russell, 2008), also identified that health visitors have a very different skill set and competency level to those of nurses as this quote from the report illustrates.

> *"They are the only group able to deal with public health, maternal mental health, child development and parenting and then have the skill to bring all*

> *functions together in a way far from the 'diagnosis and treatment' approach of most nurses".* (Russell, 2008, p3)

In a professional briefing on *The New Birth Home Visit* (Newland 2008), Newland compares the skills and knowledge provided during preparatory education programmes for nursing with that of SCPHN health visiting. It is very clear from this comparison that the standards and competences between the two are very different. These significant differences are important to understand when employing authorities may be considering using skill mix staff to conduct a new birth visit. For this reason it is essential that the new birth visit is only conducted by health visitors who have the necessary skill, competencies and training to undertake this and it is not appropriate to delegate this visit to a non-SCPHN practitioner.

Analysis and review of the competences between preparatory nursing education and SCPHN health visiting suggests correlation for just one competency in the domain of "stimulation of awareness of health needs" (NMC, 2004a) and "care delivery" (NMC, 2004b).

> **"Communicate with individuals, groups and communities about promoting their health and well-being".** (*Health Visiting*, NMC, 2004a)

> **"Consult with patients, clients and groups to identify their need and desire for health promotion advice".** (*Nursing*, NMC, 2004b)

Consideration of the content of these two domains means that it is possible to identify the key features of these competencies. In explanation, the nursing competencies prepare the registered nurse to undertake actions, for example:

> *"Collect data".*
> *"Use a range of communication and engagement skills".*
> *"Identify and respond to patients".*
> *"Use appropriate risk assessment tools".* (NMC, 2004b)

Conversely, the competencies within the SCPHN/health visitor programme prepare the health visitor to be able to undertake actions, critique information and make decisions about how to respond appropriately to the findings, for example:

> *"Develop and sustain relationships".*
> *"Collect and structure data".*
> *"Undertake screening of individuals and populations and respond appropriately to findings".*
> *"Work in partnership with others to protect the public's health and well-being from specific risks".* (NMC, 2004a)

In the case of a new birth visit is not possible to anticipate the outcome in advance of its completion (Cowley, 1995; Cowley and Billings, 2003; Houston and Cowley, 2002). It is also not possible to diagnose the mother, baby and family as "normal" before

Understanding the concept of skill mix

the health visitor has made an assessment even if the mother is having a second or subsequent baby (Cowley, 1995).

Building therapeutic relationships lies at the heart of community practice and is integral to all the work the health visitor undertakes. This relationship provides the context and is the vehicle for the work community practitioners do in partnership with parents. The knowledge and skills required to develop and sustain relationships are very different to those of the registered nurses competencies to communicate and engage with clients. Branson, Badger and Dodds (2003) have expressed concern that skill mix may affect the building of therapeutic relationships. In Unite/CPHVA's (2007) response to the Department of Health's (2007) review of health visiting, anxiety was also expressed by CPHVA members that there was insufficient understanding of the time needed to develop relationships with clients.

The 2008 Netmums Survey (Russell, 2008) also agreed with this as the following quote from the study reveals:

> *"The health visitor is unique in two respects. First, they are welcomed into the homes of parents, and if they are given the opportunity, they develop strong relationships with families that mean they are uniquely trusted. Second, when properly trained and enabled by management, they have a broad range of skills that allow them to support men, women and children in a holistic way".*
> (Russell, 2008, p3)

Managers, other professionals and commissioners of services frequently fail to understand the complexity of health visiting practice and the skills and knowledge entailed in health visiting. There is often an assumption made that a nurse can be substituted for a health visitor. For example, in conducting health needs assessments some employing authorities are now recommending these can be conducted by a staff nurse.

Evidence from Coomber *et al* (1992), mapped some of the unique cluster of skills and activities relevant to health visitors and other community nurses. These skill profiles show how similar activities compared when carried out by different grades of staff within the same team. The skills needed by health visitors to conduct health needs assessments are very different from the type of assessment conducted by nurses and midwives. Unite/CPHVA's (2007) response to *Facing the Future* (DH, 2007) reported a quote from a CPHVA member at a workshop in the South of England (who had been a midwife with 20 years' experience and was now a recently qualified health visitor) that:

> *"She didn't know how much she didn't know about health visiting before she trained as a health visitor, and that midwives do not have the competencies to carry out assessments on families".* (Unite/CPHVA, 2007, p16. Recommendation 5 Esher Meeting)

This quote illustrates the difference that exists between health visiting, midwifery and nursing. Whilst acknowledging that modern nursing roles are changing and there is a move to embed preventative health care in nursing there are still fundamental differences that separate health visiting and school nursing from generic nursing roles. From the point of view of skill mix development, clear understanding of others' roles, competencies, skills and knowledge is important if skill mix is going to work effectively and the best use made of the different and complimentary skills of other staff.

Tension and difficulties appear to arise when it is perceived that skill mix staff are being used inappropriately to perform roles for which they have not received nationally recognised training. In some employing authorities staff are receiving training and competencies in a bolt-on way rather than through properly validated and nationally recognised structured education programmes. This type of ad hoc training is often very specific-focussed on a particular goal or task and is very different from educating an individual with the necessary knowledge, skills and theory underpinning the practice. It may give rise to issues of accountability and is potentially unsafe for clients.

Unite/CPHVA's Health Visitors' Forum has produced a document on *The Distinctive Contribution of Health Visiting to Public Health and Wellbeing (Unite/CPHVA, 2008)* using the *Principles of Health Visiting* (Cowley and Frost, 2006) to demonstrate to commissioners and others what specific roles health visitors can undertake in practice, given the opportunity and adequate resources. Twelve different examples have been produced to illustrate this; they are available to download from the Unite/CPHVA website: www.unitetheunion.com/cphva

KEY POINTS

- Nursing and Specialist Community Public Health Nursing are very different forms of practice; although they have much in common there are very clear differences as discussed above.
- Other occupational groups have much to contribute to skill mix teams but it is essential that their different skills and competencies are used appropriately.
- The voice of the public and users of the service needs to be acknowledged and acted on by PCTs and employing authorities when designing services.

Rationale for introducing skill mix

There are two main driving forces behind the reasons for the introduction of skill mix:

1. Workforce issues related to spiralling staff costs and the age demographic of the workforce.
2. The increasing complexity of health care needs.

Workforce issues

In 2002 Professor Clive Booth in a review of nursing, midwifery and health visiting, predicted that there would be insufficient numbers of health visitors to deliver the public health agenda in the future. Financial deficits in employing authorities have since resulted in cuts, taking the form of frozen posts, service redesign and redundancies. This has caused confusion when the public health evidence and policy

Understanding the concept of skill mix

supports the need to increase the numbers of health visitors, school nurses, district nurses and midwives.

Health visiting has been especially badly affected. An ageing health visiting workforce, and the lack of investment in the training of new health visitors over time, has eroded their numbers forcing employing authorities to rely progressively more on skill mix. Skill and grade mix introduction has become a particular issue as the number of whole time equivalent (WTE) health visitors has dropped dramatically since 2004. Indeed, DH figures report a loss of 13.5% WTE health visitor jobs between 2004 and 2008 and recent figures from the Care Quality Commission (2009), would suggest the fall may be even greater. A survey by Unite/CPHVA (CPHVA, 2007) using the Freedom of Information Act revealed a 40% cut in the number of health visitors being trained in England in 2006. A new "Action on Health Visiting" programme has been launched by the government in an attempt to rebuild the profession (DH, 2009).

Increasing complexity of health care needs and the diversity of provision

The changing role of other health care providers will also impact on skill mix working and teams. The pattern of health care delivery has changed and is increasingly focussed on devolved care in primary care or home environments (DH, 2000; DH, 2001; DH, 2006a; DH, 2008, Darzi, 2008). The technical advances mean that people who have chronic illness and life-limiting conditions are able to live longer than ever before. Advances in foetal and neonatal medicine mean that pre-term babies have a better chance of survival and infants and children with complex health needs are being managed at home and in primary care settings. As people generally are now living for much longer there is a large increase in the over 60s population with a corresponding reduction in the number of people working and paying taxes in order to sustain the NHS and other public services. By 2021 it is estimated that 40% of the population will be over 50 (based on 2002 Government Actuaries Department population projections).

Taking these variables into account it is essential that appropriate skill mix be used to increase client services and offer a greater range of health promotion/public health activities. Skill mix could be used to align services more effectively and more appropriately to the health needs of the local population. It is possible that the right formula of skill mix could maximise human resources, reduce inappropriate expenditure and allow team members to work to their maximum professional capacity.

There is an increasing variety of different services provided by a range of professionals, para-professionals and volunteers to children and families in the community. These types of services add to the rich mix of provision that community practitioners need to be aware of, and work alongside.

KEY POINTS

There are two main driving forces behind the reasons for the introduction of skill mix:

1. The workforce issues and spiralling staff costs.

2. The increasing complexity of health care needs.

The need to introduce skill mix with care

The figure below demonstrates the impact of professionals' skill level? on children's outcomes.

Figure 1: The skill level of the professionals delivering parental programmes affects the improvement in a child's anti-social behaviour

Reaching Out: An Action Plan on Social Exclusion. HM Government 2006, p61

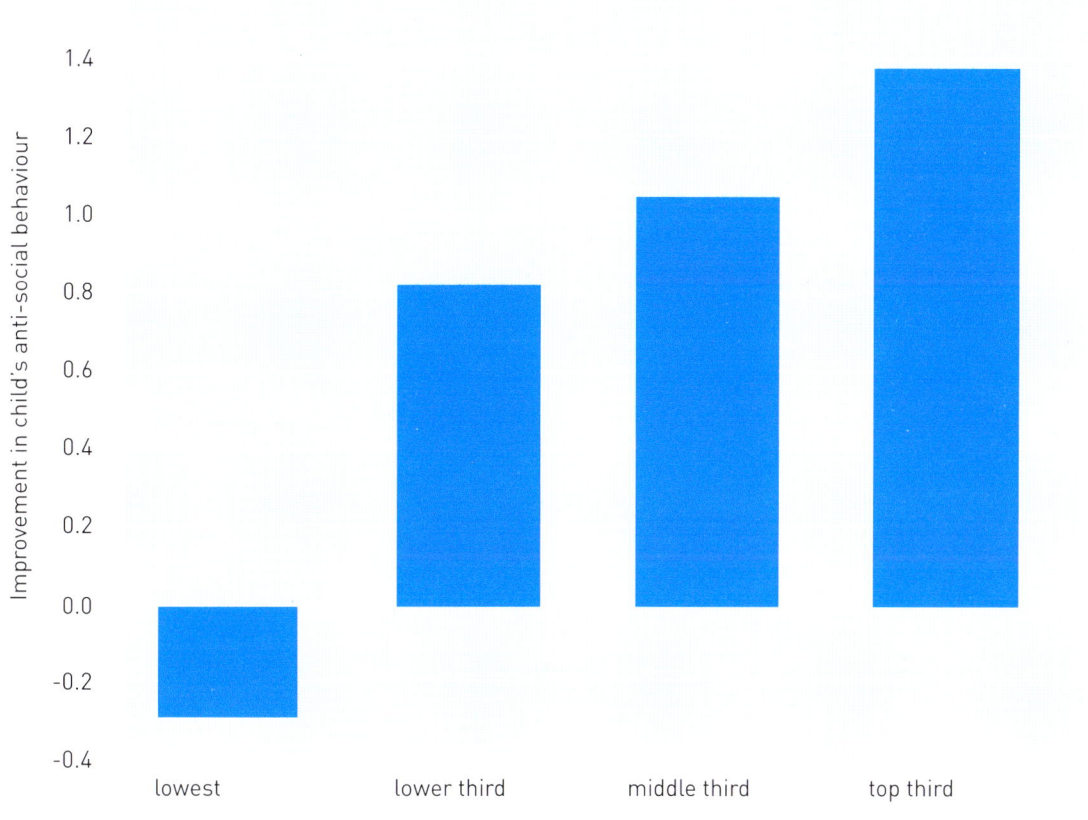

Evidence base for skill mix

There is a growing need for services to be evidence based and to be able to demonstrate measurement of outcomes. However, there is a significant lack of robust evidence concerning skill mix in community settings and it is therefore necessary to examine what evidence and models have emerged in recent years to inform practice.

There is a relative lack of recent research into skill mix, particularly in community health settings. Much of the existing work done has been as part of a local audit or an

Understanding the concept of skill mix

evaluation of service development or change rather than as a research study. Studies often had small sample sizes, poor response rates and many have not been published which limits the availability of information in the public domain. The published information is also of varying quality, rigour and sample size.

The search through the literature on skill mix in community practice however highlighted recurring professional concerns and issues over skill mix. These are summarised below:

- The difficulties inherent in practice in accommodating new skill mix roles within existing teams and the dual management structure needed to facilitate this when staff are employed by differing organisations (see the Starting Well Project, Mackenzie (2006) below.
- Skill/grade mix introduction and implementation based on an economic model of health.
- Overall increased caseload responsibility and accountability for standards and quality of care when delegating to skill mix staff or teams.
- Concerns over training for the new roles, as it is often done "on the job". This highlighted the need for adequate education as opposed to training and for quality supervision.
- Extra time was needed to adequately manage, train and develop skill mix staff on top of caseload management and responsibility.
- Accountability and delegation issues for non registered staff and NMC registrants who are not health visitors.
- Change in roles and responsibilities for health visitors and school nurses having to manage and lead skill mix staff or teams. This often requires extra training and support for SCPHNs in order to facilitate this new way of working.
- Underestimation of the time needed to manage skill mix staff or teams and supervise skill mix staff.

These broad themes are explored in more detail in the studies below and highlight the complexities and challenges of trying to manage skill mix in a community practice.

Wright (1998) analysed health visitors' activity data to determine their professional opinions of their current and ideal skill mix. The data was collected by semi-structured questionnaire and statistical returns. From a stratified random sample of 50 health visitors within a PCT, there was a 90% response rate. The sample represented urban, rural and mixed geographical areas and provided a mix of GP-attached, geographically aligned and mixed establishments that were involved in a variety of health visiting interventions.

Wright specifically highlighted the following issues:

- Overall increased caseload responsibility and accountability for standards and quality of care when delegating to skill mix staff within skill mix teams.
- Increased paperwork and liaison duties, there was an increase in workload due to the need to monitor support staff leading to a decrease in client contact. Staff felt this needed a team leader role.
- Concerns over training as most of it was done "on the job" and staff felt this was insufficient. They also identified that health visitors themselves need adequate

training to utilise skill mix effectively. Relevant quality training and good liaison were prerequisites for success.
- The majority of staff felt clerical support was the only acceptable skill mix that was non nursing.
- Staff would only accept skill mix if it was in addition to the current complement of staff.

Although this study was conducted in 1998, other recent surveys (Cowley *et al*, 2007) and the Durdle Davis Omnibus survey (Adams and Craig, 2007; 2008) reflect similar findings and professional concerns.

Mcknight (2006) explored the human resource experience following the introduction of a staff nurse role into a health visiting team and the issues and challenges that needed to be overcome. Success in this single case study was measured in terms of the activity of the staff nurse rather than health outcomes or best value. The following issues were identified:

- Low staffing levels were highlighted as a barrier to practitioner role development – a secondment was overshadowed by staffing problems and the secondment could not be extended because of staffing issues.
- The problems were easily identified – the dilemma was no-one had the time to address them.
- The difficulties of implementing the new role within an existing team and the dual management and structure needed at a practice level to accommodate this.

Mcknight (2006) concluded that there needs to be proof that skill mix is cost effective, safe and satisfactory for both users and providers before it is introduced.

The **Starting Well Project (Mackenzie, 2006)** was one of Scotland's four health demonstration projects. The Starting Well project in Glasgow used paraprofessionals, untrained healthcare support workers (HSW) from local communities, to support health visiting teams to pilot a skill mix model for health visitors working with vulnerable families. The project used a multi-method approach that examined both processes and outcomes. Two main challenges were identified:

1. Developing potentially vulnerable members of staff (to be able to work with vulnerable families)
2. Co-management of paraprofessionals by the health service and a voluntary sector organisation.

A third potential challenge of implementing a new role within an existing team, proved to be less of an issue than expected in this study. The emergent challenges in relation to skill mix from this study are:

- **Suitability of the NHS as an employer for this type of employment.** Both practitioners and managers indicated that the NHS is not suited to supporting potentially vulnerable employees. Philosophically staff agreed with the idea of using paraprofessionals, but indicated that the NHS needs to rethink employment practice in relation to employing potentially vulnerable groups. Managers and staff identified that

there was insufficient capacity to provide these workers with the level of support they required both in the recruitment process and in the employment itself.
- **Supervision of vulnerable staff.** Health visitors reported that the supervision of vulnerable staff who had their own personal problems was a burden. It was a challenge to find the time to devote to developing potentially vulnerable low skilled members of staff. Hard-pressed staff perceived that their workload increased through the employment of paraprofessionals, rather than reduced, due to the level of supervision they required. The level of staff supervision needed may outweigh the benefits.
- **Time to manage skill mix teams.** The amount of time needed to manage skill mix team members was often underestimated. Extra time was needed to prepare and delegate work activities.
- **Innovation.** Innovation is in itself time consuming.
- **Co-management of paraprofessionals.** Co-management of paraprofessionals by health sector and voluntary sector organisations created difficulties in practice. In particular ambiguities in the role definition caused difficulties. There was a communication breakdown between practice level co-coordinators and teams which led to frustration and concerns over unsafe practice. Clear lines of communication and accountability are essential for safe practice. The health support workers were exasperated at having to seek approval for their decision through two different structures.
- **Issues around using local people.** The stresses and strains of recruiting local people proved to be a challenge and caused a conflict of interest. It was questioned whether families would engage with workers living in the community, as many people actually prefer anonymous professionals.
- **Strategic aims distanced from the realities of practice.** Whilst there was satisfaction at strategic level, it was problematic for health professionals in practice. This led to misunderstandings occurring in the skill mix team, due to the absence of thorough operational planning and sharing of information. This highlights the importance of testing the implementation of the theory assumptions. Evaluation is necessary to identify practice gaps and test the model works in practice.
- **Maintaining professional boundaries.** Workers crossing the line between providing a personal service and over-identifying with family problems. Kennedy *et al's* (2005) findings from the Expert Patient Programme also highlighted this aspect when the workers own acute health problems flared up.

However positive results were:

- **The strengths HSWs can bring to home visiting practice.** Despite the challenges and variation within the HSW role, health visitors were generally appreciative of the benefits that HSWs brought to home visiting practice.
- **Good employment and training opportunities for the HSW which improved the local economy.**

Carr and Pearson (2005) used focus groups in a exploratory research study to map delegation perceptions, experiences and decision making processes of health visitors and district nurses working with skill mix in one PCT in northern England. This research suggested that community practice increases the complexity of delegation decision making. The main findings from this research are listed and discussed below.

- Exploration of delegation and decision making is an underresearched topic. There is limited knowledge on the process of making delegation decisions in skill mix, which inhibits sharing, teaching and monitoring of the inherent skills necessary for these processes.
- Delegation of established care was often in conflict with the philosophy of holistic care. The task to be undertaken cannot be used as a proxy indicator of the skills required to deliver holistic care.
- Managers and commissioners of services need to understand how working in the context of community practice, increases the complexity of delegation and decision making. There are a multiplicity of factors which need consideration; attempts to reduce these to individual skills can be perceived as a threat to the process model of care which has developed in nursing; Hicks and Hennessey (2000) also echoed this point.
- The higher cognitive skills, experience, intuition and instinct are all difficult to quantify but play an important part in delegation and decision making. As this quote from a health visitor highlights.

    "Health visiting is about being proactive, once you delegate an aspect of care to a community nursery nurse they will be responding to a situation that the health visitor has already assessed. They will respond to the situation but not necessarily pre-empt or prevent a situation occurring". (Carr and Pearson, 2005, p75)

- There appears to be some confusion surrounding the staff nurse role in the community context as this appears different to that required for the hospital setting; these differences are not explicit or standardised.
- The role of the health care assistant/support worker, community nursery nurse or community staff nurse may vary between practices depending on their individual skills, experience and the needs of the locality. This can cause difficulties in practice when the same grade may have different roles and responsibilities.
- Health visitors are enthusiastic about "appropriate" workforce development to meet the needs of the growing practice agenda as this quote illustrates.

    "We would be quite happy to have skill mix on top of health visitors hours, but it's always the other way around and health visiting hours are always taken away". (Carr and Pearson, 2005, p75)

This quote may illustrate be the crux of the matter and one of the major issues that makes skill mix introduction appear unpopular and a contentious issue.

The staff in the focus groups identified the following areas of work that skill mix would be beneficial for:

1. Clerical staff for administrative activities.
2. Community nursery nurses for play work.
3. Community psychiatric nurses for mental health issues.

- Delegation of work is affected by particular contexts rather than the task or care required such as patient/client/family situation as this health visitor explains.

Understanding the concept of skill mix

> *"With some families I'll ask the nursery nurse to go in, but with others I'll do what the nursery nurse could do, because I'm still assessing other things, or I want to give the mother an opportunity to tell me about something like a suspicion that there is domestic violence".* (Carr and Pearson, 2005, p76)

- Predictability of care was highlighted as an important consideration when delegating work within skill mix teams. This can prove hard to quantify when dealing with risk and uncertainty, which is part of the community practitioner's role and is an advanced skill. A family's' circumstances can change in between visits and they may move from being routine into requiring more support or intervention. The participants stated they would only delegate routine care, however, trying to identify what was routine and what was not, was a considerable challenge to them.
- In the community there is a lack of opportunity to directly supervise care or advice given by the delegatee in the home and that the family may not be seen by any other team member for weeks, months or even a year. Cowley *et al* (2007) suggested that in the case of new clients, and, if over a year has elapsed since a family was last seen, then the situation is not predictable. In this instance the family should be regarded as unseen and require health visitor reassessment.

McKenna's (1995) exploration of the research literature on nursing skill mix substitutions and quality of care, identified the following positive findings that correlated with a rich skill mix of highly qualified staff.

- Reduced length of stay.
- Reduced mortality.
- Reduced costs.
- Reduced complications.
- Increased patient satisfaction
- Increased recovery rate.
- Increased quality of life.
- Increased patient knowledge and compliance.

His research also looked at skill mix and quality of care in relation to staff and organisational factors. The higher quality of the skill mix demonstrated the following positive outcomes:

- Increased productivity of staff.
- Reduced staff absenteeism.
- Reduced staff sickness.
- Reduced staff turnover.
- Reduced overtime.
- Reduced costs. (McKenna,1995)

McKenna (1995) comments that:

> *"Quality is difficult to measure and most of the important effects of qualified staff are invisible to the naked eye".* (McKenna, 1995, p457)

In striking contrast to this McKenna (1995) quotes several research studies which suggest that the use of more unqualified staff leads to increased staff absenteeism, increased sick time, increased costs, reduced morale, reduced staff satisfaction and reduced quality of care. In the figure below McKenna (1995) has adapted Ovetveit's (1992) cycle of low morale to illustrate this.

Figure 2: The Low Morale Cycle

McKenna (1995) adapted from Ovetveit (1992)

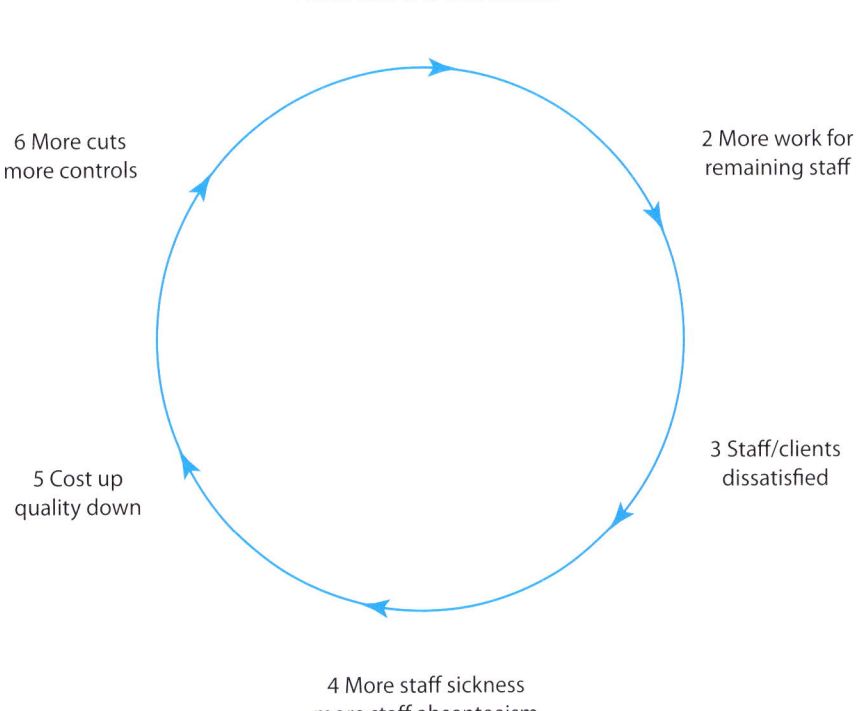

It is important that managers have an understanding of such processes and can use their knowledge and understanding of these cycles to ensure that the inappropriate use of grade or skill mix is not affecting morale, which in turn will affect the quality and safety of services provided to families.

In community practice community practitioners have struggled to try to find ways of measuring and making visible an intrinsic element of practice. In the same way care, compassion and prevention are linked to this and are difficult to measure and prove outcomes. Grifiths *et al* (2008) in an appraisal of metrics focussed on nursing and not SCPHN, identified that the patient experience of compassion is an important outcome in its own right but acknowledged the inherent difficulties there are in measuring this, as this quote reveals:

> *"Patient experience of compassionate care is an important outcome in its own right and may provide the best measure of the nursing contributions to shared outcome and evaluation of complex processes that are otherwise elusive".*
> (Griffiths, Jones, Maben, and Murrells, 2008, p24)

As in McKenna's example, most of the research on skill mix has been conducted in hospital settings which is a very different environment of care to the community.

Understanding the concept of skill mix

However, whilst the findings from hospital settings are not directly transferable to the community, it would be possible to hypothesise that similar findings could also be true for community practice.

The interesting factor that emerges from reviewing skill mix for community practice is that the focus on output may not be the best measure of outcome; it may be more productive to consider clinical input and analysis of the practitioner's role. *In Reaching Out: Think Family* (HM Government, 2007) produced by the Social Exclusion Task Force, there is a recognition that "numbers do not tell the whole story" and an acknowledgement of the genuine challenge in measuring softer outcomes *(p46)*. Soft outcomes cannot be measured directly or tangibly. Examples of soft outcomes are improved self-esteem and health awareness, empowerment, increased confidence and motivation, and the prevention of ill health, which often lie at the heart of community practice and health visiting and school nursing in particular. Ways of measuring "softer" outcomes have always presented an enormous challenge to health visitors. However the model proposed by Hicks and Hennessy (2000), outlined in Chapter 3, may offer a way of measuring softer outcomes that is more relevant for community practice.

Numerous articles have been written about nurse manpower in terms of numbers, however there has been little emphasis in the skills required and how the skill mix of the community nursing team may affect health outcomes. In the US, Olds (2002) conducted randomised controlled trials (RCTs) using "paraprofessionals" to deliver an intensive home visiting programme previously delivered by qualified professionals. The outcomes were less effective when "paraprofessionals" were used. Comparative studies are needed to see if similar outcomes can be achieved by varying skill mix combinations in community nursing teams in the UK. The ultimate aim is to provide an optimum safe service for children and families in the community. Research has shown that intensive home visiting programmes are particularly effective at reducing adverse child and mother outcomes in the most needy populations (Olds, 2006). The Health-led Parenting Support Family Nurse Partnership being piloted in parts of England is based on this research.

A Home Play project, initiated by health visitors in Sheffield (Brown, 1997) in response to locally identified need, used nursery nurse play development workers to work with disadvantaged families in a deprived area with a high number of multi-racial families. The project proved effective with positive changes for the majority and led to significant community development work. Examples such as this highlight the impact that a bottom-up approach to skill mix can have, when led by practitioners who understand the needs of their local community and are allowed to develop innovative ways of working in partnership with local people. This Home Play initiative is a practical example of the philosophy behind the *Early Childhood Development* (Irwin, 2007) quote below.

> *"The quality and appropriateness of services is a central consideration in determining whether existing early childhood development programmes improve outcomes for children".* (p10)

Irwin *et al* (2007) urge caution in the wholesale transfer of early childhood development programmes from one community to another. The authors acknowledge that whilst the principle of successful early childhood programmes may be readily transferred between settings, many will require adjusting to the social, economic and cultural contexts in which they are to be used. This is an important caveat that needs to be taken into consideration when trying to replicate successful programmes/models from elsewhere and has important implications for the establishment of skill mix working and skill mix teams. Responsiveness to the needs of the local community is central to the formation of successful skill mix development; different communities will require different staffing levels and skill mix. Universal services do not have to be uniform as illustrated in the Home Play Project (Brown, 1997). Experienced practitioners know that one size will not fit all.

Other UK schemes such as Home-Start UK – which uses volunteers to offer regular support, friendship and practical help to families who are under stress and have a child under five (http://www.home-start.org.uk/), and the Community Mothers Programmes (Suppiah, 1994) which uses lay support workers have shown to be of benefit to the health visiting service and the local community. The use of peer breastfeeding supporters, befriending schemes and other voluntary community initiatives can all add to the patchwork menu of community provision. These types of schemes offer successful examples of how skill mix can be used and its potential to enhance the health visiting service. Childrens' Centres in England now offer a plethora of staff with a range of skills which can enhance public health practice when led and managed by health visitors.

The consumer view on health visitors and skill mix

Although the focus of this section is on health visiting, where recent surveys by the Family and Parenting Institute (FPI), and Netmums have been completed, many of the messages and issues are relevant to nurses working in the community.

A parent survey of 4,475 parents conducted by Gimson (2007) for example was overwhelmingly supportive of health visitors:

> "Our results were dramatic. Parents love health visitors. They overwhelmingly want parenting and health advice from them". (Gimson, 2007, p2)

The Gimson (2007) FPI poll revealed that:

- Eighty-three per cent of parents wanted support in their home. Parents were much less keen to go to a doctor's surgery (39 %) or a children's centre (41 %).
- Seventy-six per cent wanted parenting support and advice on child health and development from a "trained health visitor with up-to-date-knowledge".
- Thirty-three per cent wanted it from a nurse (perhaps reflecting a lack of public knowledge that health visitors are trained nurses). The other interpretation of this finding could be that the majority of parents did not want to receive support from nurses, so nurses should not be regarded as a substitute for health visitors.
- Fifteen per cent from a volunteer with children of their own. This supports some use of community mothers, Home-start workers and peer breastfeeding supporters etc within skill mix teams.

Understanding the concept of skill mix

- Sixteen per cent from a child care worker (nursery nurse).
- Eight out of 10 parents agreed that *"all parents could benefit from a good health visitor who visits enough times to build up a relationship"*.

This statement concurs with the research of Davis and Spurr (1998); Jack *et al* (2005); Barlow *et al* (2005); Kirkpatrick *et al* (2007) and indicates how vital this time to build up a trusting relationship is, to both families and practitioners; a factor not easily measured or quantified in time and motion studies or recorded in activity data.

The survey by Netmums (Russell, 2008) also suggested that mothers value the traditional model of health visiting and the majority of mothers in their survey said that the most important feature of a health visitor is that she should have the *"time and willingness to listen to what I say"*.

Both the Gimson (2007) research and the survey carried out by Netmums (Russell, 2008) survey indicate that the consumer has very strong views on the service they require and value from health visitors.

Consumers and clinicians are provided with powerful levers to ensure that quality services, acceptable to the user, are provided and maintained. These include the NHS Constitution (NHS, 2009) and some of the Public Service Delivery Agreements (PSDAs). For example, in PSDA 19 (HM Government, 2007), *Ensure Better Care for All,* Indicator 1: The Self reported Experience of Patients/users, and Indicator 6, GP Services, which is concerned with increasing patient satisfaction in primary care and ensuring patients have access to services when needed. This coupled with the five pledges made in *Our NHS, Our Future, NHS Next Stage Review Leading Local Change* (2008).

Over 70 % of mothers in the Netmums Survey (Russell, 2008) stated they would prefer to have *"one health visitor who knows me and my family rather than having a mixed team, even if they were providing sound advice"*. This has implications for those PCTs who have chosen to replace health visitors with a lower grade mix team.

Parents were asked about the use of teams and corporate caseloads where they have contact with different health visitors, and staff such as community staff nurses and nursery nurses. Whilst a few mothers appreciated seeing a number of different people the majority reported that it led to two problems:

1. They miss out on building a relationship with a trusted individual who mothers then feel they can share their problems with.
2. Great variety in the advice that one family might receive.

It would appear from these large consumer surveys that parents have very clear views and preferences on skill/grade mix, team working and corporate caseloads.

The traditional model of continuing personalised care by the same health visitor, who has built up a trusting relationship with the family and has detailed knowledge of them, has often been cited as the main cornerstone of primary care and is strongly associated with client satisfaction (Davis and Spurr, 1998; Jack *et al*, 2005; Barlow *et al*, 2005; Kirkpatrick *et al*, 2007).

KEY POINTS

1. The health visiting service is delivered to undifferentiated caseloads. This is an important distinction to make and is of critical importance in determining which work can be safely delegated.
2. Responsiveness to the needs of the local community is central to the formation of successful skill mix development; different communities will require different staffing levels and skill mix. One size will not fit all – universal services are not the same as uniform services.
3. Parents value the continuity in relationship with a well educated and trained, trusted professional such as a health visitor.

2 Integrated children's services and skill mix

This chapter explores how new national standards for working with children and families are inextricably linked to the future planning of service delivery in this area and cannot be ignored. This is of particular relevance in England with the introduction of more integrated health and social care teams within Children's Centres.

Improving skills and standards within integrated children's services

Skill mix teams can form part of integrated children's services and some community practitioners are involved in leading or working in them. However these teams evolve, the drive towards improving skills and standards for those employees working with children and families will undoubtedly play a major role in the deployment of skill mix teams to provide effective, integrated services in the future.

The Change for Children Programme and the advent of Integrated Children's Community Teams 0–19 in England, which were proposed under the *Children Act* (2004), will have an impact on the future delivery of health visiting and school nursing services.

There has been a concerted effort across the UK to bring into line many of the disparate qualifications and skill sets of workers for a range of occupations. In particular there has been recognition of the need to standardise the knowledge and skills levels required by those volunteers and employees who work with children and families. Consequently, in recent years a range of qualifications and standards have emerged to help improve the quality of care in this area.

The Integrated Qualifications Framework (IQF)

Future workers within skill mix teams in England will be affected by the new Integrated Qualifications Framework (IQF). The IQF is part of the Children's Plan (DCSF, 2007), which sets out the Government's vision for children and young people and the services for them over the next 10 years. Integrating health, education and children's services as well as other providers of care for children and families, is an ambitious agenda that will require careful management and excellent professional leadership.

The IQF has been developed by the Children's Workforce Network, a strategic alliance of 12 different organisations, including the Nursing & Midwifery Council who worked closely with Children's Workforce Development Council (CWDC) The CWDC works closely with colleagues in the Children's Workforce Network (CWN) to address common issues across the whole of the children's workforce and to find answers to common challenges. The IQF will provide a set of approved qualifications that allows progression, continuing professional development and mobility across the children's workforce. It will be a comprehensive set of qualifications up to and including degrees and postgraduate qualifications that are agreed to be appropriate for people who work with children. The IQF will support shared values and learning approaches across the children and young people's workforce and reflect the *Common Core of Skills and Knowledge for the Children's Workforce* (DfES, 2005).

It is essential that the overriding principle in any joint, integrated or skill mix working arrangement must remain the development of safe joint working practices so that the workforce meets the needs of children and families and the public are protected. The valuable lessons learnt from Victoria Climbié, Peter Conolley ,(DH, 2003a, Laming 2009) and other serious case reviews must be applied, especially in relation to information sharing and workers being adequately supported and supervised. In the Victoria Climbié case (DH, 2003a), and other serious case reviews; the quality of supervision that workers receive appeared to be a critical factor in child protection work. There needs to be standards of supervision for all staff working in skill mix teams. A clear career framework and regular quality supervision is important for safe practice to ensure children are protected. Different workforces share different values and these need to be reconciled within skill mix teams. The Integrated Qualifications Framework (IQF) with the emphasis on cross-sector core units and using national frameworks is another potentially helpful way for skill mix teams of the future to be able to resolve some of the challenges outlined

These new developments will significantly alter the future education and training for all individuals who provide services to children and families. They will also have far reaching implications for all engaged in community practice and the development of skill mix and integrated working.

KEY POINTS

1. It is essential that the overriding principle in any joint, integrated or skill mix working arrangement must remain the development of safe joint working practices so that the workforce meets the needs of children and families and the public are protected. The valuable lessons learnt from Victoria Climbié and Peter Connelly (DH, 2003, Laming, 2009) and other serious case reviews must be applied, especially in relation to information sharing and workers being adequately supported and supervised in skill mix working arrangements.
2. The Integrated Qualifications Framework (IQF) is being developed by the Children's Workforce Network. It will support shared values and learning approaches across the children and young people's workforce and reflect the *Common Core of Skills and Knowledge for the Children's Workforce* (DfES, 2005). This will impact on the shape of future skill mix development and have implications for all engaged in community practice.
3. Skill mix remains an underresearched area which requires urgent investment in.

Integrated children's services and skill mix

National Occupational Standards for Working with Parents

As the range of workers who are involved in supporting parents and children grows, it is important for health visitors to be aware what level and standard of skill is expected of them. National Occupational Standards (NOS) provide a reference to assess ability of level and describe what an individual needs to do, know and understand in order to carry out a particular job role or function.

National Occupational Standards (NOS) define the competencies which apply to job roles or occupations in the form of statements of performance, knowledge and the evidence required to confirm competencies for a range of occupations including health skills. They are jointly owned by all the alliance partners within *Skills for Care and Development and Skills for Health* http://www.skillsforcare.org.uk/home/home.aspx across the UK. The standards are comprised of core units which are common to all practice and augmented by a large number of additional units which reflect specialist areas of work. It has been recognised that all agencies providing children's services should adopt common standards and all practitioners working with families and children need to have a *Common Core of Skills and Knowledge for the Children's Workforce* (DfES, 2005;).

The aim is to establish better career pathways founded on increased commonality of skills and knowledge and driven by a new national infrastructure to support the workforce development. In addition to this, other standards have been introduced which apply to all practitioners who work with parents.

Community practitioners who work with children and parents will need to have competency in both sets of standards. This has important implications for existing and future skill mix staff, as all skill mix staff will be required to meet these standards.

The development process of the National Occupational Standards (NOS) for Work with Parents and the NOS for Family Learning were funded by the DfES and supported by the Parent Education and Support Forum (now known as Parenting UK), and the National Institute of Adult Continuing Education (NIACE). These standards will have implications for all staff working with parents in any care setting.

The NOS for Work with Parents and the NOS for Family Learning were developed in conjunction with the sector and approved by the UK Regulatory bodies Qualification and Curriculum Authority (QCA), Qualification and Curriculum Authority Northern Ireland (QCA NI), Scottish Qualifications Authority (SQA), Qualifications, Curriculum and Assessment Authority for Wales (ACCAC), in April 2005. They apply to work with parents across the four countries of the UK.

The NOS for Work with Parents can be used to:

- Recognise previously acquired competences.
- Identify knowledge and skills gaps.
- Benchmark practice against the standards.
- Ensure training is relevant to job roles.
- Facilitate self-assessment.

- Help to develop and retain a more effective workforce.
- Support organisational review and planning.
- Improve recruitment.
- Enable staff to achieve through the workplace.

These NOS can bring everyone into the "learning cycle". Unlike the qualifications that are based on them, the National Occupational Standards themselves are not set at levels. They define the competence, skills, knowledge and understanding required by those who work with parents and can be used to develop and monitor these requirements in individuals, services and skill mix staff. All skill mix staff who work with parents will need to meet these standards. The NOS for Work with Parents can provide a useful tool for managers to develop skill mix staff who do not meet these standards. It can also be used by health visitors to determine activities that can safely delegated to members of a skill mix team whose qualifications comply with these standards.

Common Core of Skills and Knowledge for the Children's Workforce

Skill mix staff who work with children will be expected to comply with both the NOS for Work with Parents and the *Common Core of Skills and Knowledge for the Children's Workforce* (DfES, 2005). These common core skills and knowledge recommended for work with children are described under the following six main headings:

- Effective communication and engagement with children, young people and families.
- Child and young person development.
- Safeguarding and promoting the welfare of the child.
- Supporting transitions.
- Multi-agency working.
- Sharing information.

It is anticipated that having a common core of skills, knowledge and competence for the widest possible range of workers in children's services, including volunteers, this would support the development of more effective and integrated services. It would introduce a common language amongst professionals and support staff, so starting the process of breaking down some of the cultural and practice barriers within the children's workforce. The future emphasis will be on skills rather than individual roles.

KEY POINT

1. The NOS for Work with Parents can provide a useful tool to develop skill mix staff who do not meet these standards. These together with the introduction of the Integrated Qualifications Framework and the *Common Core of Skills and Knowledge for the Children's Workforce* (DfES, 2005) will influence present and future skill mix staff and training.

Integrated children's services and skill mix

It is expected that, over time, everyone who works with children, young people and families will be able to demonstrate a basic level of competence in the six areas of the *Common Core of Skills and Knowledge for the Children's Workforce* (DfES, 2005). The government envisages that the *Common Core of Skills and Knowledge for the Children's Workforce* will form part of qualifications for those working with children, young people and families and it will act as a foundation for training and development programmes run by employers and training organizations.

Both the NOS for Working with Parents and the *Common Core of Skills and Knowledge for the Children's Workforce* (DfES, 2005) will have implications for future nurse education, SCPHN training, community nursery nurse training and for all members of the primary care team who work with children and families. It is possible that, in the future, the NOS for Working with Parents and the Common Core of Skills and Knowledge will be integrated into every person's job description involved in this field. Competency could be demonstrated through the use of personal development plans.

> There is now a health care assistant (HCA) toolkit which was developed by the Working in Partnership Programme (WiPP) in collaboration with Staffordshire University, available from: http://www.rcn.org.uk/development/hca_toolkit

When considering the introduction of skill mix or reviewing existing skill mix teams it is important to consider the NOS for Working with Parents and the *Common Core of Skills and Knowledge for the Children's Workforce* (DfES, 2005) to ensure all staff are up to date and will meet the required standards.

KEY POINTS

1. Community practitioners who work with children and parents will be required to have competency in both the *Common Core of Skills and Knowledge for the Children's Workforce* (DfES, 2005) and the National Occupational Standards for Work with Parents. This has important implications for existing and future skill mix teams, as all team members will be required to meet both sets of standards.
2. When considering the introduction of skill mix or reviewing existing skill mix teams it is important to consider the NOS for Working with Parents and the *Common Core of Skills and Knowledge for the Children's Workforce* (DfES, 2005) to ensure all staff are up to date and will meet the required standards.

Standards for Better Health

Standards for Better Health, published by the Department of Health in 2004, sets out the standards that all health care organisations in England should be achieving. It identifies 24 core standards within seven domains that all NHS health providers in England should achieve, and a further 13 developmental standards that they should be working towards achieving. These core and developmental standards cover all aspects of health, including the safety of patients, clinical effectiveness and cost effectiveness, so they are important to consider when planning changes in the way services are to be delivered using skill mix. They also apply to any independent health providers who are commissioned to treat NHS patients. The Care Quality Commission is responsible for the monitoring and inspection of these standards in which it assesses a trust's quality of care and how well it is complying with the core standards and the steps it is taking to meet the developmental standards. All staff involved in skill mix working should be aware of these standards and how they may relate to the work/care environment they are involved in.

The developmental standards are designed to provide a framework for NHS trusts to deliver services that continue to improve in line with patients' increasing expectations. These standards were originally introduced in 2004 by the Healthcare Commission (now the Care Quality Commission); they have now produced separate criteria documents, one for each type of trust (i.e. acute and specialist services, mental health and learning disability services, ambulance services, and primary care trusts). In 2007/2008 the criteria for assessing core standards for primary care trusts (PCTs) were set out as "elements" for each of the core standards and cover seven core areas of activity listed below (*Criteria for Assessing Core Standards in 2007/2008 Primary Care Trusts*, Healthcare Commission, 2007*)*.

The seven core domains:

1. Safety of patients.
2. Clinical effectiveness and cost effectiveness – is it providing treatment in line with national guidelines and in the most effective way?
3. Governance – is it well run?
4. Patient focus – does it organise its services around the needs and preferences of patients?
5. Accessible and responsive care.
6. The care environment and amenities.
7. Public health – does it improve, promote and protect the health of local people?

Within each of the core domains above are a number of core standards and developmental standards related to that domain. For example in the domain of safety there are four core standards and one developmental standard. Staff who work in primary care and who are involved in managing skill mix staff may like to reflect on the above core domains and consider them in relation to the daily work and measure how well they feel they perform. This may provide a useful tool for staff to evaluate the services they provide and they may like to ask patients/clients on their views and experience of the services provided.

The following core standard has been highlighted as central to much of the work that health visitors and school nurses are involved in:

Core Standard 2 is the domain of safety and states "*Health care organisations protect children by following national child protection guidance within their own activities and in their dealings with other organizations*".

Integrated children's services and skill mix

The Care Quality Commission (CQC) has regional and national safeguarding leads for both children and adults. They have a helpline anyone can ring if they are concerned over safeguarding standards, complaints are taken very seriously and are investigated, As a result of enquires made to the helpline, the Care Quality Commission may decide to carry out spot checks on a PCT or employing authority. This is an additional useful resource for community practitioners to be aware of if they have concerns over the safety of patients/clients or governance issues and feel that their concerns are not being addressed within their employing authority. It is worth examining the 24 *Core Standards for Better Health* (2004) as they can be a powerful tool in ensuring acceptable levels of safety and care.

> The CQC helpline number is **03000 616161.** Their website is at: http://www.cqc.org.uk/guidanceforprofessionals/contactcqc.cfm
>
> Email: enquiries@cqc.org.uk Practitioners can look at any PCT and see how compliant they are with the core standards. PCTs are also expected to comply with the Joint Area Review (JAR) staying safe element which they are also monitored on annually.
>
> The Health Care Inspectorate Wales (HIW), a department of the National Assembly for Wales, is responsible for inspecting and investigating the provision of health care by, and for, Welsh NHS bodies. Since 1 April 2005, HIW has also been responsible for the regulation of the private and voluntary health care sector in Wales, having taken over this role from the Care Standards Inspectorate for Wales. Their website is http://www.hiw.org.uk/

In 2009 the Healthcare Commission changed its name to the Care Quality Commission and is now part of a wider inspectorate, however, its inspection function continue. The new Care Quality Commission will not have a role in individual complaint handling. two-tier system is in place and complainants who remain unhappy after local resolution will have the option of taking their case to the Health Service Ombudsman.

Equivalent bodies to the Care Quality Commission in Scotland and Northern Ireland, respectively, are NHS Quality Improvement Scotland and the Health & Personal Social Services Regulation and Improvement Authority Their web addresses are http://www.nhshealthquality.org/nhsqis/CCC_FirstPage.jsp and http://www.rqia.org.uk/home/index.cfm respectively.

In considering the quality of care given by skill mix teams it is important for managers and practitioners to be aware of the standards expected of those team members and the potential consequences not only for patient safety, but also for the possible consequences of not adhering to the standards expected of them. It is therefore imperative that in developing skill mix teams that there is a clear assessment of client need and a matching of that need to the skills of employees which are now more easily recognised as a result of the increasing emphasis on the standardisation of qualifications required in this field of practice.

KEY POINT

1. The CQC will investigate concerns of staff regarding client safety which NHS staff feel haven't been adequately addressed by their management.

3 The realities of skill mix in the workplace – issues for professionals in practice

This chapter explores a range of professional issues which are relevant to NMC registered practitioners in how skill mix is deployed in practice. These include issues of professional regulation, accountability, delegation, information sharing, confidentiality and informed client consent. There is an in-depth examination of the implications of skill mix for NMC registrants and the factors that can affect delegation in community practice.

Professional regulation

Potential changes in inter-professional regulation and emerging roles need to ensure quality, safety and public protection through the regulation of services and the professions (DH, 2007a; Longley *et al*, 2007; DH, 2007b). Consideration needs to be given to the sharing of the regulatory role between statutory regulators and employer. Reviews of professional regulation (DH, 2006a; DH, 2006b), highlighted the need for clarity over the respective responsibilities of local employers, local commissioners and professional regulators to ensure high professional standards, competence, and conduct. The abuses of the GP Harold Shipman, nurse Beverly Allitt and others, ha focussed media, public and professional attention on regulation issues and public safety.

Safeguarding Patients (DH, 2007b), was the Government's response to the recommendations of the Shipman Inquiry's fifth report and to the recommendations of the Ayling, Neale and Kerr/Haslam Inquiries. *Safeguarding Patients* (DH, 2007b) should be read in conjunction with the Department of Health White Paper (2007a) which deals with similar issues from the perspective of professional regulation. This White Paper (DH, 2007a), proposed bringing the regulation of health professions more in line with one another. However, responsibility for standards in nurse education will remain with the Nursing & Midwifery Council (NMC). Strengthening professional regulation for all health professions has recently been a key focus for government (DH, 2007a; DH, 2007b). At the time of writing the regulation of healthcare assistants is under discussion and this could also have implications for community nursery nurses

It is important that the health care professionals of the future are well trained to be able to work safely and effectively with others to meet the needs of the communities and the population they serve. All health care practitioners will need to have the requisite skills, competencies, and knowledge to fulfil the role, lead the team and ensure safe and appropriate delegation and supervision of the workforce. This is a separate issue to that of regulation but important to consider in relation to skill mix and public safety.

The changing nature and structure of health care delivery and the implications of devolution across the four countries of the UK all have to be considered. Scotland, Wales and Northern Ireland are also addressing the quality agenda in ways that meet the needs of the populations that they serve and that are suited to the way their health care systems are organised. The DH White Paper (2007a) recognised that the proposals in the two reviews of professional regulation (DH, 2006a; DH, 2006b) would need to be adapted in order to work well in Scotland, Wales and Northern Ireland. Future arrangements need to enable health professionals to move easily around the UK during their careers. These future developments may affect how skill mix evolves across the UK.

The Bologna Process underpinned by the Bologna Declaration (1999, European Higher Education Area), aims to make quality assurance standards more comparable and compatible throughout Europe. The Bologna Process is supported by Ministers of Education from 29 European countries including the UK and aims to align higher education qualifications and nursing across Europe; this will influence the way in which nurse education evolves in the future. With the increased mobility of health care staff nationally it is vital that there is alignment of qualifications to ensure public protection.

The Sector Skills Council for Social Care, Children and Young People and the introduction of the Integrated Qualifications Framework for the Children's Workforce across the UK will also impact on the future of nurse education, post registration training and skill mix. Members of the Children's Workforce Network, of which the NMC is a member, are discussing how to create public sector skills pathways, joining up local government health and social care nationally. This could change the way future community health and social care services are delivered and significantly alter the way skill mix is developed in the future. Skills for Care and Development comprise: the Care Council for Wales, Cyngor Gofal Cymru

CCW or CGC, the Northern Ireland Social Care Council (NISCC), the Scottish Social Services Council (SSSC) and Skills for Care.

KEY POINTS

1. Led by the NMC and Department of Health a major review of pre and post registration nursing has taken place which will affect the way skill mix evolves in the future.
2. Work is taking place to strengthen professional regulation for all health care professions.

Accountability

To be accountable means one is answerable to someone for something, or some action, or failure to take some action, one should have done. This implies that the practitioner should be able to explain the rationale behind the decisions that they take. Accountability cannot exist without responsibility being granted and accepted. Bergman's (1981) figure below shows the pre-conditions that lead to accountability.

The Nursing & Midwifery Council (NMC) is the professional body that all NMC registrants are professionally accountable to. The core function of the NMC is to establish standards of education, training, conduct and performance for nursing and midwifery and to ensure those standards are maintained, thereby safeguarding the health and well-being of the public.

All NMC registrants, in addition to their professional body, also have a contractual accountability to their employer and are also accountable in law for their actions. Lines of accountability for NMC registrants are considered in more detail below and in Figure 4 (p39).

> *"As a professional you are personally accountable for actions and omissions, in your practice and must always be able to justify your decisions. You must always act lawfully, whether the laws relates to your professional practice or personal life. Failure to comply with this Code may bring your fitness to practise into question and endanger your registration".* (NMC, 2008)

Figure 3: Model of the Pre-conditions Leading to Accountability

Bergman, 1981

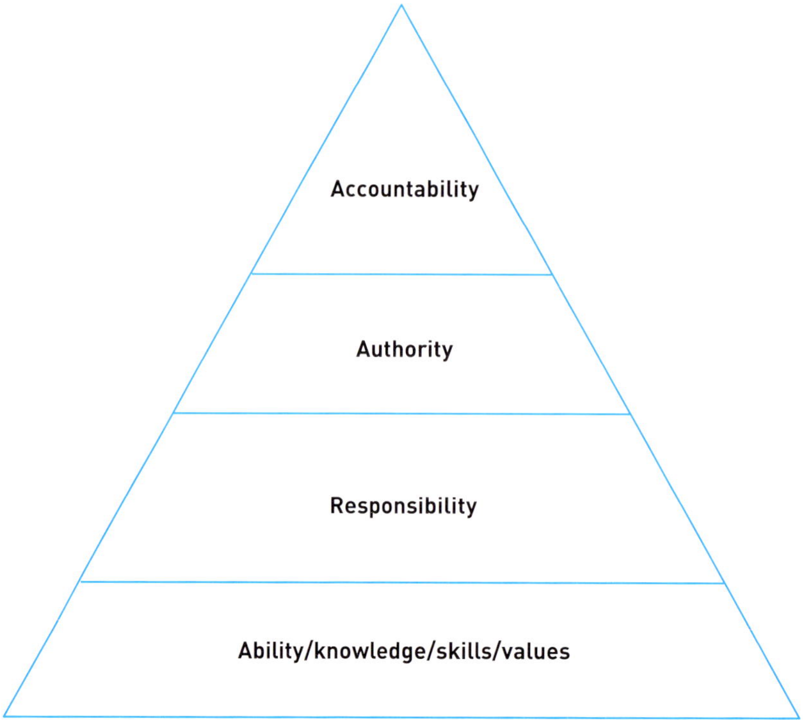
Accountability
Authority
Responsibility
Ability/knowledge/skills/values

Accountability is an integral part of provision to practice. In practice registrants have to make professional judgements in a wide variety of circumstances. Professional accountability is fundamentally concerned with weighing up the interests of patients and clients in complex situations. In practice the NMC registrant must use their professional knowledge and skills to make decisions; they must be able to justify their decisions, omissions or course of action and be able to show that the decisions they took were in the best interests of the patient or client.

Non-registrants may be required to carry out care delivery not delegated by a registrant because it is part of their terms and conditions of employment; this appears to becoming increasingly common in team working, grade and skill mix situations. In this case the employer sets out competencies to be met and should also accept "vicarious liability". Registrants supervising in such cases although not accountable for the non-registrant's actions are accountable for ensuring the care delivered is safe and within the agreed parameters of their competence. In these situations the employer becomes accountable for that delegation. The NMC registrant will however continue to carry responsibility to intervene if he/she feels that the proposed delegation by the employer is inappropriate or unsafe. The decision whether or not to delegate an aspect of care and to transfer and/or to rescind delegation is the sole responsibility of the NMC registrant and is based on their professional judgment. Advice on delegation for nurses and midwives is available from the Nursing & Midwifery website: www.nmc-uk.org

For example, if a NMC registrant is supervising a nursery nurse in a skill mix team who may be employed by another employer in a Children's Centre, she is not accountable for the nursery nurse's practice. The nursery nurse is accountable for this to her employer and in law either by criminal prosecution or civil claim. However, an NMC registrant is accountable if she fails to take action if an individual is perceived by the registrant not to be competent to perform her role, or the registrant fails to intervene to prevent her from continuing to do something that is, unsafe, inappropriate or incorrect.

A manager supervises all staff but is not accountable for their practice; however the manager has a duty of care to the public, her staff and is accountable to her employer (and professional body if she belongs to one), for their decisions, actions and omissions. Health service providers like all public bodies are accountable to both the criminal and civil courts to ensure that their activities conform to legal requirements.

Accountability is demonstrated to clients through:

- Record keeping.
- Confidentiality.
- Informed client consent.

Each of these issues should be considered when setting up a framework of accountability with skill mix staff.

When considering skill mix it is important to remember that NMC registrants are accountable for actions and omissions. For example, if they do not agree with an employer who tells them to delegate specific activities to junior practitioners but still go ahead and comply even though they may believe that in doing so the client may suffer harm. They are accountable for their decision to comply with their manager's request and cannot use the excuse that they "were only doing what they were told by management". This is not a defence in law or in terms of fitness to practice in line with the NMC code of professional conduct.

The NMC registrant must take action through the correct channels to inform the employer that they will not do it, why they will not do it and what alternative action they have taken to ensure the patient/client remains safe.

Accountability issues can become very challenging when NMC registrants are managing many skill mix staff or holding caseload responsibility for large numbers of children or families. Gimson (2007), under the Freedom of Information Act (2000), researched the numbers of whole time equivalent (WTE) health visitors who work with children under five and revealed that:

- Fifty per cent of health visitors in the poll had caseload responsibility for more than 300 children.
- Twenty-two per cent took charge of more that 500.
- In one PCT health visitors had caseload responsibility for over 1000 children.

This is clearly unsafe and unacceptable; an NMC registrant would be advised to take action through the correct channels that were outlined in the accountability section.

At the CPHVA Conference in 2006 it was revealed by a Cornish school nurse to the then Health Secretary, Patricia Hewitt, that she had a caseload of over 9,000 children which Patricia Hewitt described as "horrific" (Unite/CPHVA, Press Release, 2007). These increasingly occurring types of scenarios draw urgent attention to the need for clarity over caseload responsibility. Unite/CPHVA recommends an absolute maximum caseload of 400 children and an average of 250 children for a full time health visitor, regardless of the presence of corporate working or skill mix. This should be less in areas of deprivation and where there are high numbers of vulnerable families (Unite/CPHVA website http://www.unite-cphva.org/ The Annual Omnibus Survey (CPHVA Omnibus, 2008), commissioned by Unite of 1,000 randomly selected health visitors, also reported that in England 40 % of health visitors had responsibility for 500 children. Seventy-two per cent of the health visitors surveyed revealed that their workloads and levels of responsibility had also increased and they also had to manage and coordinate skill mix teams. Stress levels had consequently risen with 76 % reporting an increase in stress. If the health visitor is managing additional workers who are not NMC registrants and/or is the only SCPHN managing a caseload the accountability and responsibility associated with this is very high. Should this lead to the practitioner experiencing increased levels of stress, she should inform her line manager as her employer has a duty of care to her in terms of her physical and psychological wellbeing.

Vicarious liability

Vicarious liability means that the employer is accountable for the standard of care delivered and is responsible for those employees working within areas of competence

Skill Mix in Community Nursing and Health Visitor Teams: Principles into Practice

appropriate to their abilities. To remain covered by an employer's vicarious liability clause an employee must only work within their abilities and sphere of assessed competence within the policies and protocols of an employing authority and their contract of duty. The NMC Code (2008) recommends that all NMC registrants take out professional indemnity insurance and ensure they are clear about their insurance status; it is advisable to check whether additional arrangements need to be made.

The NMC advises that local policies should be developed or amended using this information. The *NMC News* provides regular updated information sheets on the website.

Lines of accountability

Registered nurses have four different lines of accountability:

- To the public.
- To the client.
- To the employer.
- To their professional body (NMC) as illustrated by Andrews (1995) in Figure 4.

Depending on the type of incident that occurs, an NMC registrant could face action in all of the four areas illustrated below. An extreme example of this was NMC registrant Beverly Allitt who was struck off the register and sentenced to life imprisonment after killing four children and injuring a further five. The most common reason for staff being disciplined is in relation to record keeping.

Figure 4: Lines of Accountability

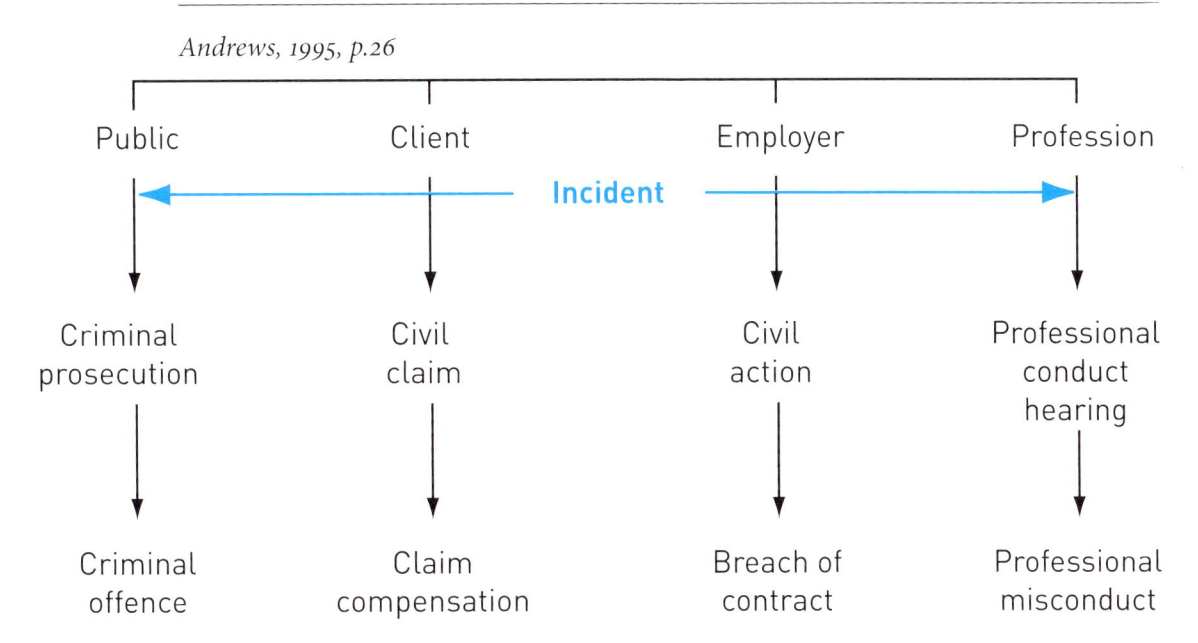

Andrews, 1995, p.26

Public	Client	Employer	Profession
←	Incident	→	
Criminal prosecution	Civil claim	Civil action	Professional conduct hearing
↓	↓	↓	↓
Criminal offence	Claim compensation	Breach of contract	Professional misconduct

Examples of lines of accountability in practice are the training, protocols, procedures and policies that employers are required to have in place to protect employees and the public. The employees are accountable and responsible for attending mandatory training, reading, understanding, following and applying the set policies, procedures and protocols in practice. The employer is responsible for ensuring adequate, accessible training is available and that policies, procedures and protocols are in place and are regularly updated to protect the public and the employee.

Examples of this include:

- Attending regular manual handling courses to ensure safe moving and handling practice.
- Attending training on infection control to protect the public and staff.
- Accessing annual safeguarding training to ensure they are up-to-date and familiar with the national and local policies and procedures for safeguarding children and vulnerable adults.

Much of this essential training should be provided as part of the employer's induction programme and annual or bi-annual updates which are required to ensure safe practice. Attendance at mandatory training is an area that is audited when staff have their annual appraisal.

All staff who have contact with children must be checked by the Criminal Records Bureau (CRB). The purpose of the CRB check is to reduce the risk of abuse by identifying candidates who may be unsuitable to work with children or other vulnerable members of society. This is an essential requirement for all staff working with children and families and it is the responsibility of the employee to ensure these are kept up to date.

It is essential that clear lines of accountability are established from the beginning and that all skill mix staff are aware of the safeguards that exist to protect the public. All skill mix staff who are NMC registrants, and non-regulated skill mix staff, need to be fully aware of how their accountability relates to the other staff they work with and who may be accountable for the actions or omissions of others. Non-regulated members are accountable to the public, the patient and the employer within their sphere of ability and responsibility. All registered nurses have the same lines of accountability as shown in Figure 4 (p39).

Ability

Ability relates to competence to undertake the task or role and to having the appropriate knowledge, skills and attitude. Skill without knowledge, understanding and the appropriate attitude does not equate with competent practice. Thus, competence is *"the skills and ability to practice safely and effectively without the need for direct supervision"* (UKCC, 1999; Watson 2002). McFarlane (1986) states that *"practice without theoretical basis becomes a ritualized performance, unrelated to the health needs of individuals and society"*. Part of this ability relates to monitoring and assessing changes in health and providing information so individuals can make decisions regarding their own health and the practitioner can facilitate and encourage action.

Competence

Competence is an individual's ability to apply knowledge, understanding, skills and values within a designated scope of practice. This is demonstrated in practice by the effective performance of that specific role and an understanding of its related responsibilities. Competence implies that the individual can critically reflect on their practice, and adjust and improve their practice as a result of this reflection. What is deemed to be good practice usually rests on a consensus view shared by other professionals and professional bodies. The NMC (2008) has defined competence as:

> *"a bringing together of general attributes – knowledge, skills and attitudes. Skill without knowledge, understanding and the appropriate attitude does not equate with competent practice. Thus, competence is 'the skills and ability to practise safely and effectively".* (NMC, 2008)

The above definitions of competence relate closely to Bergman's (1981) bottom tier of the accountability triangle shown in Figure 3 (p36).

The challenge for community practitioners is the need to consider how their professional accountability and responsibility for skill mix staff may be managed, whilst they are engaged in a wide range of professional duties, in an environment that is much more variable and less "controlled" than that of a hospital or health centre. The complexity of the delegated task and the stability and predictability of the patient/client health status and family situation are further dimensions that need to be considered when deciding to delegate an aspect of care.

Responsibility

Accountability and responsibility are different. Responsibility is the process of being responsible for something and implies an authority to act and take decisions independently. Responsibility implies knowledge of the requirements of practice and relates to undertaking the task or role in accordance with training protocols and within the framework in which the practitioner has been asked to work. Responsibility implies an understanding of professional accountability in relation to this. The NMC (May 2008), define responsibility as:

> *"A form of trustworthiness; the trait of being answerable to someone for something or being responsible for one's conduct".* (NMC, 2008)

When delegating to others the registered practitioner has a responsibility to ensure they have determined the knowledge and skill level needed to perform the delegated task for that client/patient in their service setting. This is discussed in further detail in the section on delegation.

Authority

Accountability comes with **authority** to act, to decide what should be done and to be answerable for that decision. It implies autonomy to make decisions about care based on a higher level of skill and knowledge and the ability to respond to changing care situations within the scope of the role. For example, the chief executive of a PCT or employing authority has accountability, authority and responsibility in terms of service provision for that organisation. There is real concern currently that professional autonomy and authority is being eroded as the role of the health visitor is increasingly prescribed by her employer rather than as a result of her/his professional judgement. This compromises their professional accountability.

In practice authority is the NMC registrant's right to make decisions and implement them based on their professional knowledge, competence and judgement. There may be a conflict of interest between what an employer expects or requires of an individual and a professional's code of conduct, performance and ethics, particularly if health resources are limited. In these cases an NMC registrant is bound by The Code (NMC, 2008), to consider what is in the client's/patient's best interests; all other factors are secondary to this. The NMC registrant has a duty to safeguard the client/patient and must act immediately to manage any risk. They are duty bound to inform someone in authority if they encounter problems that prevent them working to their Professional Code (NMC, 2008), or other nationally agreed standards. They are required by the NMC (2008) Code to report their concerns in writing if they identify problems in the environment of care, which are putting people at risk.

Whatever decisions or judgements are made the registrant must be able to justify their actions and clearly document them.

KEY POINT

1. If NMC registrants are concerned about the safety to clients of delegating a specific activity, they are advised to consult local policy and also discuss the matter with a senior colleague or manager. Managers have a responsibility not only to their staff but also to the patients/clients in the care of their staff. The NMC Code of Professional Conduct (2008), provides guidance on a NMC registrant's responsibility. When faced with a professional dilemma the first consideration must be the safety of patients/clients and what is in their best interests.

    Any manager who is an NMC registrant may be required to justify their actions if inadequate resources seem to affect the situation. Managers who fail to act appropriately when informed of environments of care that could potentially endanger patients/clients could face local disciplinary action and fitness to practise proceedings by the NMC if they are an NMC registrant.

Unite/CPHVA advise practitioners to visit the NMC website and download the latest A-Z sheets on delegation for NMC registrants and other relevant advice sheets on accountability, environment of care, risk management, whistle blowing and the other essential advice sheets. This will enable them to fully comprehend their duty of care and responsibilities.

Employing authorities and commissioners of services face considerable challenges over their accountability. Cowley and Andrews (2001) identified that there is a need for greater clarity over the accountability of SCPHNs for those clients they have caseload responsibility for, but may not have seen for a period of weeks, months or even years. The SCPHN remains accountable because she has made a decision not to see the client. However, if this is not a decision based on professional judgement but the outcome of not having sufficient time then the SCPHN is accountable for taking action to keep the client safe i.e. informing the employer and complying with the employing authority's clinical governance procedures and risk assessments. This can complicate the delegation or allocation of work to skill mix staff if a child/family/patient has not been seen for some time. Following best practice the SCPHN or senior staff member would be required to assess the family before they could delegate the work to a junior grade of staff.

Dilemmas in health visiting practice often relate to the level of service that ought to be available and by whom it should be provided. If a service is available in a locality, access to that service is often determined by the health professional and their clinical judgement. This can make delegation decisions more complex in skill mix teams as both the care environment and changes in family circumstances or health can be unpredictable.

Cowley and Andrews (2001) examined health visitors' accountability and the employer's duty of care in various examples from practice. Using different case scenarios to analyse various dilemmas, it was apparent that the legal requirement was for the delivery of care to be of an acceptable standard. Lack of facilities or lack of resources provided no legal defence for the professionals concerned. Cowley and Andrews (2001) also considered the significant accountability issues that arise in practice for health visitors who hold caseload responsibility. In the four scenarios presented, two important issues arise:

1. The significance of a "health visitor's professional judgement" which places a large onus of responsibility upon the individual health visitor.
2. The importance of determining what constitutes an "acceptable standard of practice" particularly in terms of provision for the population for whom the health visitor has responsibility. Decisions about what counts as an "acceptable standard" depends, not only upon an individual practitioner or Trust determining what kind of practice they will offer, but also upon what is considered reasonable by the whole profession. The legal requirement is for those delivering care to meet an acceptable standard. Lack of facilities or lack of resources does not provide a legal defence.

Unseen families pose the highest risk to the PCT or employing authorities; anyone not seen for a year or more must be regarded as unseen and as such would require an assessment by a health visitor. The impact of a reduced health visiting service and increase in skill mix staff needs to be considered in terms of the continuing

CASE STUDY

A health visitor received a letter from the Human Resources manager. The letter advised the health visitor that an investigation will be held relating to a number of allegations of professional misconduct. The allegations are:

- That the practitioner failed to contact four children in need/child protection families in breach of the trust's policies and national legislation.
- Record keeping for a number of families was in breach of the trust's policies and the NMC guidelines on *Record Keeping*; (NMC, 2007).
- Failure to establish contact with child protection families meant that those clients did not receive the appropriate level of service in accordance with local policies and national legislation.

The health visitor was suspended on full pay pending the outcome of the investigation. The investigation gathered evidence from the health visitor and members of the team and found that there was a case to answer under the trust's disciplinary procedure.

What happened at the health visitor's disciplinary hearing?

The evidence presented at the hearing included: documentation relating to the families for which the health visitor had responsibility; witness statements from members of the health visiting team including the team leader and the child protection adviser; and a statement from the health visitor.

The defence offered by the practitioner is based on the circumstances which made it difficult for her to carry out the work. She did not deny that she had not undertaken the family visits or completed the record keeping. Her defence was that workload pressures prevented her from prioritising this work and she had delegated some duties to the community nursery nurse but these were not carried out. In her evidence, the health visitor was unable to demonstrate that she had alerted her line manager to these difficulties, nor could she demonstrate that her workload was excessive. She believed that the nursery nurse should take some of the responsibility for the situation.

The decision of the disciplinary panel was to dismiss the health visitor for gross misconduct for her professional misconduct. She appealed unsuccessfully and the employer reported her to the NMC.

What lessons can be learnt from this example?

Most importantly is the need to recognise the responsibility the practitioner has to all clients and the authority that has to be exercised to prioritise work on the basis of need in accordance with established policies and the legal framework. Whilst an excessive workload has to be addressed, this can only be done by ensuring management is made aware and help and support are provided. In this case there was no evidence of excessive workload and the attempt to delegate work inappropriately to the community nursery nurse was a significant act of misconduct for which the health visitor was fully accountable. It represented a failure in her professional authority and recognised that she remained accountable for her decisions, work and professional standard.

responsibilities held by the employing authority. The duty of care may revert to the GPs, provided he/she is informed, if the health visiting services are reduced to the point at which caseload responsibility stops being a manageable alternative. However this decision should be taken at a senior management level when all attempts to resolve the resources issue had been exhausted. Community practitioners with caseload responsibility need to be mindful of their accountability and legal obligations to ensure safe standards of practice are maintained (see Unite/CPHVA Fact Sheets on *Determining Optimum Case Load Size* and *Managing Safely and Guidelines for Managing Vacant Caseloads,* Unite/CPHVA, 2007).

The NMC reported in June 2006 that 13 % of the total monthly enquires to the Professional Advisory Service (PAS) were for information and advice regarding staffing levels and appropriate skills, this figure is higher for Unite/CPHVA. The NMC advises registrants to be aware of and to implement both local and national policies and legislation regarding the delivery of care.

Delegation

> **Delegation** is the transfer to a competent individual, the authority to perform a specific task in a specified situation that can be carried out in the absence of that nurse or midwife and without direct supervision (NMC, 2008).

When community practitioners delegate tasks that are normally within their normal practice they usually retain accountability for that person's care, and must therefore continue to ensure the delegated duties are carried out properly and delegation remains appropriate. This presents a greater management and supervision challenge in a community setting than it does in the more controlled environment of a hospital or clinic. Accountability for professional decisions and conduct relates directly to the authority that a practitioner has. Every practitioner has full responsibility for her/his actions or omissions.

In a skill mix situation the lines of accountability can sometimes become blurred. For example, when being told to delegate certain tasks to a junior skill mix member of staff, the senior practitioner will not have the authority to make the decision about who does what in terms of the restructure/structure of the team. However the delegating practitioner will have the authority to make decisions about their actions and omissions i.e. the decision to delegate the task will be theirs.

When delegating to a junior member of the skill mix team the two key questions the NMC registrant practitioner needs to consider are:

1. Is the delegatee competent to carry out the task?
2. Does the delegatee believe she is competent to carry out the activity?

   The decisions about who is available to delegate the task to, is not theirs (in this situation) and often they do not have the authority in many situations to make this

The realities of skill mix in the workplace – issues for professionals in practice

decision as it is dependent on the team structure and availability of skill mix staff. They need, therefore, to be clear about where their line of accountability lies.

The reverse is also true for example when the NMC registrant is happy that the task can be delegated to a junior member of the skill mix team. The NMC registrant is accountable and responsible for this decision and needs to be able to justify the judgment in terms of the reasons/information that they have used to make this decision e.g. they have observed the person doing the task, and have discussed this task with the person and outlined what needs to be done. Furthermore, the delegatee has then been checked by questioning/discussion to ascertain that she has understood what needs to be done and how it needs to be done. This checking process also needs to acknowledge that the person knows what to do and who to access if something happens that is unexpected. The delegating NMC registrant is also accountable for obtaining an update about the task – was it done and what the effect/outcome was. It is not sufficient to offer in defence that the senior person who was delegating the task merely assumed that it would be/was done.

Examples to illustrate delegation in practice are described on pages 48 -50.

All employers in the NHS must be satisfied that their NMC registrant employees' professional conduct meets the standards required within the workplace and established by the NMC's Code (2008). This, in effect, means that NMC registrant practitioners can be held to account and may be subject to investigation and disciplinary action where there are concerns about their professional conduct.

Principles for delegation when working with skill mix

The overriding factor that must be addressed in relation to delegation is whether this is in the best interests of the patient or client. All other factors follow on from this key issue. When a community practitioner delegates work to another person, competency issues must be addressed. It is imperative for those delegating care and those employees undertaking delegated duties that they do so within a robust local policy framework to protect the public and support safe practice. The delegating practitioner needs to consider the following:

- Is the work at an appropriate level for the delegatee to undertake?
- Does the person have the knowledge and skills to be able to do the work?
- Is the scope and parameters of the work to be carried out clearly understood?

The delegatee practitioner is then accountable for that work. The person delegating the work is accountable for checking that it has been done. This can prove problematical in community settings when staff are working unsupervised in people's homes. The skill mix member of staff, once they have agreed to do the task, is responsible for undertaking the task or role assigned to them and completing the requirements outlined at the outset. Clear lines of communication and the process for reporting back must be established. Each case is unique and should be assessed before a task can be delegated to ensure that it is in the patient's best interests at the time. This can pose dilemmas in the community when a family may not have been seen for some time. It is important that community practitioners are confident to delegate appropriately and also to refuse to delegate if they believe it is not in the client's best interests. The NMC registrant has the right to refuse to delegate if they have clear evidence to believe that it would be unsafe to do so or if they are unable to provide or ensure adequate supervision (see NMC website for advice sheet on delegation for registered nurses and midwives).

To prevent potential problems the following principles should be adopted when delegating work:

Planning and preparation	• Clear measurable objectives need to be set so they can be identified as done or not done for the episode of care to be delegated. • Dates for reassessment should be set at the beginning, together with plans of action if the client situation changes. • Planned lines of communication and feedback need to be identified and sufficient time dedicated to ensure they are followed through. • Risk assessments should be made to ensure the health and safety of all skill mix staff are considered and appropriate action taken. Issues related to personal safety and home visiting need to be addressed for all skill mix staff and appropriate training given. • Written protocols should be developed which identify action to be taken when untoward or unpredicted occurrences take place; this must include a time response clause (see *Managing Safely factsheet*, Unite/CPHVA, 2007). • Appropriate training in these areas should be developed and made available to all skill mix staff; this training needs to be ongoing.
Day-to-day management	• Clearly identified action plans if the client situation changes. • Good supervision is important in ensuring less skilled staff are supported and gaps in skills or service provision are identified. • All staff who have delegated responsibilities must have immediate telephone access (within 4 hours) to a senior colleague for emergency advice and support. Protocols must, in particular, be specific regarding Friday afternoon contacts and last day of term contacts for school health teams. • A lead person should be identified to ensure continuing evaluation of the skill mix and highlight/lead changes when indicated. • All these actions should be adequately resourced. In particular dedicated time is needed to ensure practitioners are able to lead skill mix staff in a manner that enables them to exercise their accountability properly. Clear objectives for the scope of delegated work need to be agreed alongside the implementation plans that have been negotiated and agreed with the client and the skill mix staff.

Review and maintenance	• A regular system of supervision and appraisal needs to be in place for all skill mix staff. This should feed into professional development plans. The outcome of supervision and appraisal systems should have authority within the organisation to ensure that appropriate professional development and training identified is undertaken. This will include mandatory training in child protection and safeguarding. • Clinical supervision is a key tool in ensuring appropriate and safe practice. It is vital that all skill mix staff have planned supervision sessions on a regular basis. For school nurses and their skill mix staff this should be a minimum of one hour each half term. This is especially important when less skilled staff are undertaking episodes of care in complex environments in particular where there are potential child protection issues. Where skill mix staff are being managed by people who are not NMC registrants, a suitable clinical supervisor must be identified.

The NMC Code for Standards of Conduct, Performance and Ethics (2008), provides the following guidance on delegation and risk management that NMC registrants need to be mindful of when delegating to skill mix staff:

KEY POINTS

To delegate effectively:

- You must establish that anyone you delegate to is able to carry out your instructions.
- You must confirm that the outcome of any delegated task meets required standards.
- You must make sure that everyone you are responsible for is supervised and supported.

To manage risk:

- You must act without delay if you believe that you, a colleague or anyone else may be putting someone at risk.
- You must inform someone in authority if you experience problems that prevent you working within this Code or other nationally agreed standards.
- You must report your concerns in writing if problems in the environment of care are putting people at risk. (NMC Code, 2008, p4)

NMC registrants are advised to check the NMC website regularly for updates.

Examples of delegation in practice

Below are two descriptions of the sort of delegation issues that could occur in practice. The first is when the health visitor might decide not to delegate an episode of care and the second when the health visitor decides to delegate an episode of care using the principles outlined above.

A mother attends clinic and specifically approaches a health visitor she knows for some advice about her toddler's diet and eating habits. Whilst discussing this, she then confides that she is concerned that she may also have an eating problem as she has started to make herself vomit in order to manage her own food intake. However she does not want this information sharing with other family members at present, but does want help with it. Normally the policy, following the corporate caseload protocol, is that the visit would be allocated back to the team and the community nursery nurse would follow up to give general advice on the toddler's diet. However, in this case there are concerns about the wellbeing of the mother who had specifically approached the health visitor that she had developed a trusting relationship with after the birth of her previous baby.

This example highlights some of the complexities that can arise in community practice and the importance of building trusting relationships with clients. In this case the mother approached a health visitor she knew and trusted about her toddler's diet and eating habits. It was then possible for her to be able to share her own concerns over her own eating pattern. The health visitor would need to follow this family up and deal with both the toddler and mother's eating habits. The health visitor in this example felt it was in the client's best interests not to delegate care to any other practitioner. The health visitor would need to make a full assessment of the situation in partnership with the parent and agree what future support and care this family may require. It would not be appropriate or in the client's best interest to delegate this visit to a nursery nurse, even though she could advise on the toddler's diet and eating habits. It may be appropriate in the future for the nursery nurse to become involved with helping to support the family over the toddler's diet if the parent is in agreement with this.

The next example illustrates appropriate delegation to a community nursery nurse.

A health visitor has been working with a family and feels the mother requires additional help and support in promoting play activities with the child. This would be an appropriate delegation as the nursery nurse has the necessary knowledge and skills in relation to child development and is able to relate this knowledge to the play requirements of a child at a specific age. The delegating health visitor will need to confirm this competency and check that the nursery nurse is able to deliver this care in the specific environment (i.e. in a client's home, to work alone) and can document and record the outcome and work to the agreed care plan.

The health visitor will also need to confirm that the nursery nurse is able to record and document the outcome and process of the care episodes. The nursery nurse is not accountable to the NMC or a professional body because they are not a registered profession. However, they are accountable to their employer, the public and their colleagues. This is different to the line of accountability for a nurse registered on the NMC register.

The SCPHN is accountable for delegating the task – i.e. accountability is for this action and they are responsible for making provision for the task to be done and what to do and who to contact if there are unanticipated developments. The SCPHN is not accountable for the actions of the nursery nurse. The nursery nurse who has accepted the task is responsible for doing it in the correct way. Once they have accepted the task, they are responsible for it. The SCPHN is accountable to the extent of being able to justify why and how they made the decision to get the other person to do the task (i.e. this is their line of accountability). The delegating professional is responsible for confirming that the task has been done and for reviewing and assessing the effect/outcome and the care plan, and ensuring that the nursery nurse has regular clinical supervision to ensure appropriate and safe practice.

It is important that all delegating professionals understand their accountability for their actions and omissions and their line of accountability. It is important to be clear that they are not accountable for the actions of another but they must be able to justify their decision to delegate a task to another person. When delegating care the delegating practitioner retains overall responsibility for that client/patient's care.

All team members must only take on work they are competent to do (i.e. have the knowledge and skills) and which is within the scope of their practice. Relevant protocols should be in place to ensure practice is safe and appropriate for all staff. For example, in the instance within a small skill mix team when the health visitor is absent due to sickness, annual leave or study day, the community nursery nurse is left without an NMC registrant; there should be clear guidance on what the community nursery nurse should do on such occasions and who will provide cover.

Factors affecting delegation in skill mix and community practice

Carr and Pearson's (2005) focus group identified four facets to delegation in relation to skill mix and the care environment:

1. Decision making.
2. The delegator-delegatee relationship.
3. Patient/client need.
4. Structural and contextual facets.

1. Decision making

Confidence in the delegation and decision-making process is an important aspect for the delegator. They need to feel satisfied that the patient/client/family needs have been assessed accurately so that delegation feels safe and is in the best interests of that person. This could result in a longer assessment process before delegation occurs.

2. The delegator-delegatee relationship

The delagator/delagatee relationship is affected by how well known the delegatee is to the delegator and the former's level of competencies. Any lack of knowledge of these factors results in reluctance to delegate or a dilution in delegation and is closely linked to accountability issues. Under the NMC Code of Conduct (NMC, 2008), NMC registrants are legally bound and accountable for their delegating decision making. Two highly valued characteristics in the delegatee were to "know their limits" and be prepared to "ask for help" when it was needed. As this quote from the study reveals:

> *"You do occasionally get a person who is a bit overconfident and thinks they can do things they shouldn't".* (Carr and Pearson, 2005, p77)

3. Patient/client need

A cornerstone of safe and successful delegation was realising that it was preferable to say to a client *"I can't deal with this I will have to refer back to the health visitor"* even though by doing this the health visitor had to make a visit to the family which could be seen as undermining delegation on a time allocation basis. However, the overriding consideration and the NMC registrant's accountability relates to what is in the client/patient's best interests; all other considerations are secondary to this.

4. Structural and contextual facets

Structural and contextual facets are also concerned with accountability. In this study Carr and Pearson (2005) identified the varying availability of the delegates especially when team members are shared between practice teams and/or work part time as a major factor that affected delegation decision making. Other constraints identified included the lack of continuity and consistency of care. Geographical distances and often the problems associated with contacting staff once they have left the office could also be problematical and inhibit delegation opportunities. The accountability issues with this are discussed in the accountability section. The context rather than the task or care required can affect the delegation such as when the health visitor feels that there may be an underlying issue such as domestic violence which she wants to give the mother an opportunity to discuss. This is an example of the highly skilled intuitive work that health visitors are educated to recognise as it relates to hidden and unmet health needs which often take time to emerge.

Two other factors emerged as important in the delegation decision rationale from this research. These could be divided into distinct categories:

1. Convenience-driven decisions based on a pragmatic approach dictated by the staff who are available rather than who is the most appropriate person to respond to this client/patient. The types of skills and care needed were not central to the decision, but geographical convenience, economic impact in terms of travel costs and practitioner time were. Another example of this was redistribution of a caseload to even out workload or cover absences and sometimes the sheer necessity of having to delegate to someone of a lower grade due to limited availability options. This finding is not driven by what is in the client's best interests but is driven by resources and an economic model of service delivery. To comply with the NMC Code (2008), practitioners would be required to follow the steps on pages 36–40 to ensure they fulfil their accountability duty.
2. Specific decisions made with the explicit purpose of responding appropriately to client/patient need. Delegation practice was related to effectiveness and economics in terms of who had the best skills and knowledge base to respond to this particular client/patient. Both the district nurses and health visitors gave examples of skill and need matching in which another worker such as a community staff nurse, community nursery nurse of health care assistant provided a combination of care over a set time period.

Carr and Pearson's (2005) study identified the complex process involved with making delegation decisions in skill mix and substitution as well as the lack of knowledge that existed in this area. These authors examined in detail the challenges for district nurses and health visitors when delegating routine or assessed patient/client need. The study respondents identified that the evolving nature of patient/client need and the unpredictability of care created difficulties in delegation. This was heavily influenced by the diversity and quality of the staff they could delegate to. It was felt essential to explore and assure themselves of the competence of the delegatees before engaging in delegation; this was a particular issue when bank or temporary staff were used. To comply with the NMC Code (2008), this is an essential requirement for all NMC registrants who are delegating work to skill mix staff. They have to ensure they discharge their accountability duty and consider patient safety and their best interests.

The majority of community care takes place in unsupervised settings, notably in people's homes, schools or other care environments. As well as the crucial issues of competence and accountability there are a number of other issues relating specifically to community practice that need to be considered when delegating care:

1. Predictability of care

The nature of home-based work requires that care delivery be fluid. Community practitioners may do a home visit with one set of objectives but find a different situation on arrival, which will mean revising their original objectives. Cowley (1995) has discussed this at length in an article entitled *In Health Visiting a Routine Visit is one that has Passed*. Predictability of care can be a real challenge when delegating work to skill mix staff, as there is little research based information to predict which borderline cases in safeguarding, developmental delay or postnatal depression will improve without help and those that may dramatically deteriorate without timely skilled intervention.

In practice the most serious cases are the ones that are the most documented and tend to be the ones that are more predictable. In the field of prevention and in health visiting in particular proving your intervention has prevented an event occurring or deterioration of a situation/condition has always been one of the greatest challenges. There is a significant shortage of simple tools to measure such outcomes. A similar situation exists when offering a 'drop-in' service to children and young people in schools or community settings. There is no way of knowing what concerns a young person will bring to the session. Similarly, in an open access child health clinic setting it is impossible to predict what concerns a parent may present with; for this reason health visitors need to be available at child health clinics to deal with such situations.

2. Developing relationships

The work of health visiting and school nursing is governed by the *Nursing & Midwifery Code of Conduct Performance and Ethics* (2008), which advises NMC registrants:

> "You must recognise and respect the contributions that people make to their own care and wellbeing". (NMC, 2008, p3)

This partnership approach has been hailed as possibly more effective in improving child health than much of the routine work done by health visitors (Goodwin, 1991). There has been a great deal of research carried out on the health visitor client relationship highlighting the need for health visitors to work in partnership with clients. This research has given us an insight into the kinds of relationships that are necessary for positive outcomes for families (Luker and Chalmers, 1990; Davis and Spurr, 1998; Cowley, 1991; De La Cuesta, 1993; Collinson and Cowley, 1998; Normandale, 2001; Brocklehurst *et al*, 2004; Barlow *et al*, 2005; Jack, DiCenso and Lohfeld, 2005; Kirkpatrick *et al*, 2007).

Bidmead and Cowley (2005 have defined this relationship as follows:

> *"Partnership with clients in health visiting may be defined as a respectful, negotiated way of working that enables choice, participation and equity, within an honest, trusting relationship that is based in empathy, support and reciprocity. It is best established within a model of health visiting that recognises partnership as a central notion. It requires a high level of interpersonal qualities and communication skills in staff who are, themselves, supported through a system of clinical supervision that operates within the same framework of partnership".* (p208)

This is the kind of relationship with clients that health visitors and school nurses might well aspire to and ideally would be able to develop given time. It will always be the most vulnerable clients who require the time to overcome their lack of trust and start to build such a relationship with the health visitor or school nurse. Developing relationships over time with clients and families may lead to them asking for additional information and help, uncovering hidden unmet needs or expressing new needs.

In *A New Vision for Mental Health* (The Future Vision Coalition, 2008), concern is expressed over the concept of "personalisation of services" as it implies it is something which is done to service users by the system rather than reflecting a move towards "self determination" and a system of support built by the individual and their advocate to help them achieve their ambitions and goals. This self-determination philosophy enables service users to choose their own route to recovery with appropriate support as needed. This self-determination model is similar to the partnership model as described above where the client retains the power and the practitioner works in partnership with the client. The *New NMC Code of Conduct* (NMC, 2008), quoted above reflects this notion, as does recent government policy (DH, 2001; DH, 2006a; DH, 2006b; DH, 2008). A common professional concern for many SCPHNs is the potential impact that introducing skill mix may have on developing and establishing this therapeutic relationship with clients.

3. Communication

Due to the unsupervised nature of community work, it is important to acknowledge the need for good communication and feedback between skill mix staff and other professionals involved. Indeed excellent communication skills are a requirement for building partnership relationships with clients as well as with staff and other agencies. Being able to actively listen and respond with empathy are key skills.

With the increasing use of the corporate model of health visiting, clients have contact with different health care professionals and skill mix staff and subtle nuances in their behaviour or interaction may not be easily noticed. Therefore, changes in service delivery need to acknowledge that these subtle communication cues may be missed or an exploration of the benefits, challenges and drawback of corporate working in health visiting and public health nursing teams (see Brocklehurst and Adams, CPHVA, 2004).

4. Ongoing nature of care

The ongoing nature of care over time means clients' needs are constantly changing. This is particularly important for ensuring public protection when less skilled staff may not pick up cues related to new needs. A one-off assessment is not sufficient and repeated assessments are a fundamental part of each contact. Cowley (1993) identified that health service managers and commissioners of services often assume that "assessment" is an activity which occurs once, and is not an ongoing process. This can present a real challenge in managing skill mix staff and in corporate working as discussed above. It also ignores the complexities of identifying who should be regarded as a "client" in a family situation. For example, the 7–8 month developmental check is an assessment and an activity that can competently be carried out by a community nursery nurse. However, in practice, this contact is used to carry out a developmental assessment a holistic family health assessment including an assessment of maternal mental health, and to promote good health practices such as in home safety and immunisation. Delegating part of the task to another skill mix staff member results in fragmentation of care and service delivery. Similarly, the annual health assessment of looked-after-children is not a "tick box" affair, but a holistic assessment by a skilled school nurse to ascertain the health status, knowledge and skills of the young person.

Delegation and record keeping

The person delivering the care must sign the entry that they have made in the client's record. The registrant is only able to sign the record if she has either given the care or has observed the care being delivered. It is not a legal requirement that all entries made by a junior skill mix staff member are countersigned. The practice of counter-signing for another practitioner who delivered the care is incorrect and unsafe practice (Newland, 2007, Newland 2007a). However, practitioners need to be aware that it is good practice to outline what measures there are in place to promote client safety when delegating care to other team members. For example, good practice would entail the provision of clearly written care plans, the instruction to the practitioner and the processes in place to ensure the worker's competence to deliver care as well as the mechanism for giving and receiving feedback. It should be clearly documented how feedback is to be given and received, and the strategy for reviewing progress of the treatment and care plan and the process for updating the care/treatment plan (, Newland, 2007, Newland, 2007a). The NMC Record Keeping and notes FAQ (2009), have provided further clarification on record keeping for pre-registration student and health care support staff (HCSS) outlined below.

> *"If you delegate the task of record keeping to pre-registration students of nursing or midwifery, or to HCSWs, you must ensure that they have the knowledge and skills to carry out this task, and that they are properly supervised. If the student or HCSW is not yet considered competent in keeping records – an opinion that may have been voiced in their performance assessments for example – then you must countersign their entries, either in writing or electronically. You have*

a duty to ensure that records completed by students or HCSWs under your supervision are clearly written, accurate and appropriate." (NMC, 2009)

The NMC Record Keeping and notes FAQ (2009) advice for delegation to non-regulated health care staff and students:

"If you delegate duties to members of the multi-professional health care team who are not registered practitioners, you are responsible for ensuring that these tasks are carried out to a reasonable standard".

Although you will not be accountable for the decisions and actions taken by the delegated person, you will be responsible for the overall management of the person in your care. You will also be accountable for your decision to delegate.

KEY POINT

Skill mix and record keeping
The person delivering the care must sign the entry that they have made in the client's record. The registrant is only able to sign the record if she has either given the care or has observed the care being delivered. It is not a legal requirement that all entries made by a junior skill mix staff member are countersigned. The practice of countersigning for another practitioner who delivered the care is incorrect and unsafe practice (*Record Keeping & the Law,* Newland 2007, Newland 2007a.).

Information sharing

Information sharing must be done in a way that is compatible with the Data Protection Act (HM Government, 1989), the Human Rights Act (HM Government,1998), and the common law duty of confidentiality. However, practitioners have a legal right to share information when it is in the best interest of the child or adult client. Practitioners are advised to keep up to date with the latest *Information Sharing Guidance for Practitioners and Managers* (HM Government, 2008) available at the web link below to ensure they, and the skill mix staff they work with, are aware of their responsibilities in this matter. http://www.everychildmatters.gov.uk/informationsharing

Record keeping systems and information sharing need to be examined and the following issues addressed when skill mix staff are employed.

1. Who has access to the record? Does every skill mix staff member need to read all the records and have full knowledge of the client or family? There will be occasions when parts of the family history should be shared (for example, there may be health and safety issues), and other occasions when skill mix staff may not need to know everything. This judgement needs to be made by the senior or the person delegating parts of care. If a skill mix member of staff is caring for the client then they will need to have access to the records. The NMC (2007) *Record Keeping Guidance* and *Record Keeping & the Law* (Newland 2007,, 2007, Newland 2007a), support the principle of shared records in which all health care team members make entries in a single record

and in accordance with agreed local protocol. The record should be consecutive, written with the client's involvement where practicable, and completed as soon after the event as possible (*Record Keeping & the Law*, Newland, 2007, Newland 2007a). Skill mix staff should not hold separate clinical records from that of the NMC registrant or other professional. Each member of the health care team's contribution should be seen of equal importance (see *Record Keeping Guidance for Nurses and Midwives* and *Record Keeping: Notes and FAQ* (NMC, 2009); *Community Nursery Nurses, A Voluntary Code of Professional Conduct* and *Community Nursery Nurses Professional Guidelines* (Unite/CPHVA, 2007).

2. A contract with a client should identify how records are kept and who has access to them. The practitioner must inform the client about the records that are kept, the rationale for keeping them, who has access to them and that they are stored in a secure, locked place – and that information is shared on a-need-to-know basis. The principle of openness and partnership with clients in this respect should be explicit.

The Caldicott Standards provide a code for good practice based on the principles of the Data Protection Act (1989). The six Caldicott Principles set out below govern how personal information is shared within the health service and local authority children's services.

> **The Caldicott Principles: a Code for Good Practice for Skill Mix Staff**
>
> 1. Justify why you need personally identifying information.
> 2. Don't use personally identifying information unless it's necessary.
> 3. In every case use the minimum amount of personally indentifying information.
> 4. Only those who need to know personal information should have access to it.
> 5. Everyone should be aware of their responsibilities with regards to personal information.
> 6. Everyone should understand and comply with the law.

In addition to the Caldicott Principles, the *Information Sharing Guidance for Practitioners and Managers* (HM Government, 2008), suggests the following seven golden rules for information sharing which are useful for all staff to bear in mind.

Seven golden rules for information sharing for skill mix staff

1. **Remember that the Data Protection Act is not a barrier to sharing information** but provides a framework to ensure that personal information about living persons is shared appropriately.
2. **Be open and honest with the person** (and/or their family where appropriate) from the outset about why, what, how and with whom information will, or could be shared, and seek their agreement, unless it is unsafe or inappropriate to do so.
3. **Seek advice if you are in any doubt,** without disclosing the identity of the person where possible.
4. **Share with consent where appropriate** and, where possible, respect the wishes of those who do not consent to share confidential information. You may still share information without consent if, in your judgement, that lack of consent can be

overridden in the public interest. You will need to base your judgement on the facts of the case.
5. **Consider safety and wellbeing.** Base your information sharing decisions on considerations of the safety and well-being of the person and others who may be affected by their actions.
6. **Necessary, proportionate, relevant, accurate, timely and secure.** Ensure that the information you share: is necessary for the purpose for which you are sharing it; is shared only with those people who need to have it; is accurate and up-to-date; is shared in a timely fashion, and is shared securely.
7. **Keep a record of your decision and the reasons for it** – whether it is to share information or not. If you decide to share, then record what you have shared, with whom and for what purpose.
(Taken from *Information Sharing Guidance for Practitioners and Managers,* HM Government, 2008, p11)

> Further details on record keeping can be found in the NMC's *Record Keeping Guidance for Nurses and Midwives,* (2009); *Record Keeping: Notes and FAQ* (NMC, 2009), and *Record Keeping & the Law,* Newland 2007, 2007), *Record Keeping and Documentation* (Newland, , 2007a).

Confidentiality

Confidentiality issues need to be considered within these information sharing principles. The client should be part of a process that establishes ground rules for who knows what aspects of both the family/client situation and the care intervention that is planned. For example, at the practitioner's first contact with the client, a broad overview of the team including how information is shared within that team should be made explicit. In addition the client should be aware that information disclosed to one member of staff may have to be shared with another. This can cause dilemmas within school nursing when information sharing may not be appropriate or realistic when working with children and teenagers in school. The setting and client group the practitioner is working with will determine how confidentiality issues are addressed. The ability to obtain information whilst respecting the client's confidentiality is essential. This is very clear in safeguarding children but there may be greyer areas of practice, see some typical examples from practice in the case scenarios below.

All skill mix staff need to be prepared and trained in how to deal with information given to them by a client but which they feel they cannot keep confidential. These potential situations should also be discussed with clients as part of the ground rules and professional boundaries. It should also be explained that the outcomes of specific episodes of care will be reported back to the professional who is senior and accountable for the overall care of the family/patient. Skill mix staff may need a fuller briefing for example if there are child protection issues, or in relation to domestic abuse and violence.

All staff working within the NHS are also bound by the NHS *Confidentiality Code of Practice* (DH, 2003), which covers the following:

- Concept of confidentiality.
- High level description of main legal requirements.
- Consent.
- Disclosure models.
- Confidentiality decisions in practice

Further information on this can be found at: http://www.dh.gov.uk/prod_consum_dh/groups/dh_digitalassets/@dh/@en/documents/digitalasset/dh_4069254.pdf

Case scenario examples to illustrate confidentiality issues

The following examples have been used with permission from The Health Informatics Service at http://www.this.nhs.uk/)

Health visiting example

A community nursery nurse is visiting a family to discuss weaning with a family, when the parent mentions that she can't eat or cook certain vegetables as they bring back unhappy memories of her childhood and a past abuse she suffered. The community nursery nurse tries to gain further details but the mothers states she cannot discuss it as it is too upsetting for her.

Questions

- What should the community nursery nurse's response be to the mother regarding the information she has disclosed?
- What should the community nursery nurse do with the information she has been given?

Children's Centre example

Dad comes into the Children's Centre reception and asks to see any information that is held on his child. You know that the parents are not married and think that they may have recently split up.

Questions

- Does the father have the right to be told this information?
- How should he request it?
- Who has parental rights where parents are not married?

School nursing example

A 14-year-old girl has been receiving contraceptive advice from the school nurse (and a supply of condoms). Her mother wishes to meet with the school nurse to discuss her daughter's treatment.

Questions

- Does the nurse have to discuss the daughter's treatment with the mother?
- What would she have to decide before agreeing to do so?
- At what age can a child be assumed to be competent to make their own decisions?

The above examples represent typical situations that occur daily in practice and illustrate the complexities of practice and the skills and knowledge community practitioners need to have *Informed client consent*

All health visitors, school nurses and community practitioners aim to work in partnership with clients. This implies the client understands the role of the practitioner and accepts the range of services being offered. The health visitor or community practitioner has a duty to be active in ensuring that this is the case and that the client has all the appropriate information to give informed consent. If another member of staff undertakes an episode of care with that client/family it is incumbent on the lead practitioner to obtain informed consent for that intervention. However, in some situations this may be unrealistic for instance when working with children and young people in school. The context, setting and client group will influence the consent issue.

Obtaining informed consent would include giving full information about the role and skills of the new worker and the objectives and possible limitations of the intervention. The client would need to consent to record keeping and confidentially issues as above. Established feedback mechanisms for clients should be clear and transparent and reviewed regularly with all skill mix staff.

4 Introducing skill mix

This chapter identifies best practice in creating and developing skill mix models and protocols in health and social care. There is a particular focus on skill mix in community care settings and some of the challenges associated with this, particularly for specialist community public health nursing (SCPHN), and the implications of skill mix in relation to safeguarding children and vulnerable adults. There is also an outline of some general principles for achieving success when introducing skill mix in practice.

Models

In this section three different models will be explored. The first model, Buchan and May (2000), consider external constraints and output. The second model by Hicks and Hennessy (2000), emphasises the clinical input and the practitioner's own subjective analysis of their role. The third alternative, proposed by Adams and Lungden (2000), is similar to Buchan and May's (2000) change model cycle but stresses that greater attention should be paid to the organisational changes and human resource management that form part of such changes, for example when skill mix is being introduced. A significant theme emerging from the literature on skill mix is the relationship between how people management is undertaken within trusts/employing authorities and the approach to skill mix implementation.

For skill mix introduction to be successful it is essential that everyone affected by the changes is consulted and involved in the process. If skill mix is imposed, problems often arise. A prerequisite for introducing and implementing skill mix is a supportive effective management who fully understand the change management principles and the stress associated with the introduction of skill mix.

The skill mix cycle based on clinical output

Buchan and May (2000) describe a change cycle which has been adapted by the author to help consider the questions and issues that need to be addressed before skill mix is introduced. Some of these questions are in the frequently asked questions (FAQs) section at the back of the book on pages 77-78. The skill mix cycle described in Figure 5, is not dissimilar to various models of managing change.

This four-stage skill mix cycle should not be regarded as a "one-off" isolated event, like any evaluation cycle it should be a continuous process to monitor the impact the changes have made.

Skill Mix in Community Nursing and Health Visitor Teams: Principles into Practice

Figure 5: The Skill Mix Cycle

Adapted by Fisher (2008) from Buchan and May (2000)

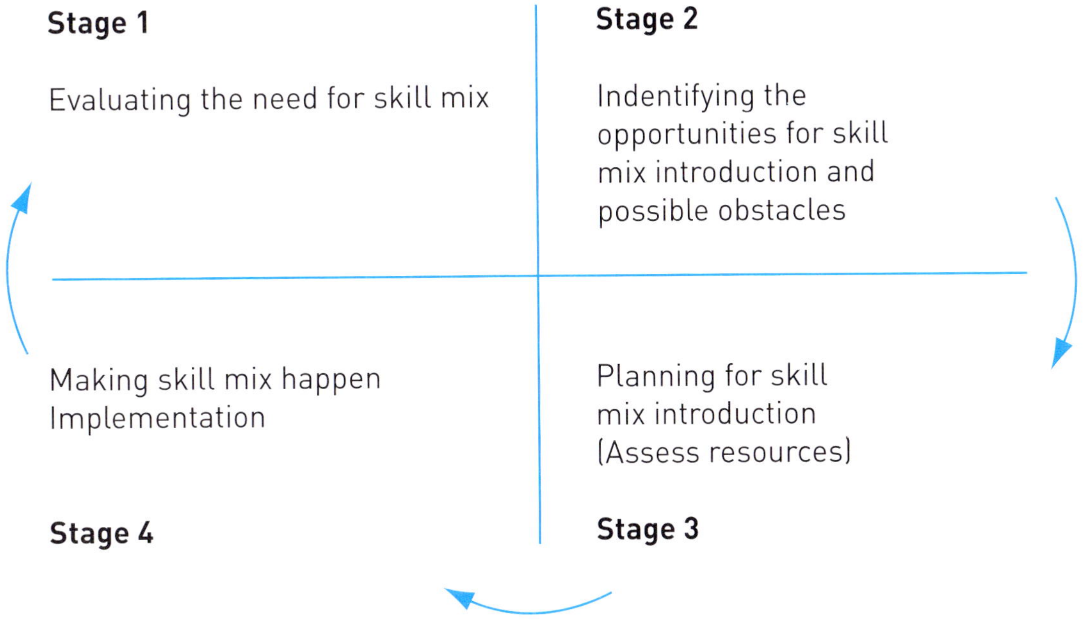

Stage 1	**Stage 2**
Evaluating the need for skill mix	Indentifying the opportunities for skill mix introduction and possible obstacles
Making skill mix happen Implementation	Planning for skill mix introduction (Assess resources)
Stage 4	**Stage 3**

STAGE 1

When introducing skill mix the current service provision needs to be examined and the following points considered. In order to evaluate the effects of introducing skill mix there needs to be clarity about the starting point with baseline indicators:

1. Needs of the client/patient groups.
2. Current level of service provision, activity levels, workload, caseload analysis.
3. Activities performed/roles and skills of the staff.
4. Quality of care provided.
5. Outcome indicators.

Stage I requires an in-depth evaluation of the need for skill mix. Current service provision needs to be mapped and defined. A detailed assessment needs to be undertaken to identify the areas in which skill mix could be safely used.

STAGE 2

This involves identifying the opportunities for skill mix introduction based on an assessment of the following:

- National pay structure.
- Staffing norms/staffing ratios.
- Employment regulation – public sector fixed allocation of jobs.
- Regulation of health workers.
- Autonomy of education sector.

Introducing skill mix

- Accreditation of organisations.
- External control of budgets.
- Statutory/voluntary/private mix of skill mix provision.
- Labour market factors (relative pay, job and pay protection, *Agenda for Change* etc).
- General economic situation.
- Societal/cultural values.
- Risk assessments need to be done to ensure public protection and safety of staff.
- National and local policies and protocols.
- Professional regulation and guidance on best practice.
- Public service delivery agreements and statutory guidance.
(Adapted from Buchan and May, 2000)

Job roles and descriptions must be based on the needs of the service users and they need to be reviewed and updated regularly to ensure they are in line with the *Agenda for Change* (AfC), job evaluation process. Unions and other professional organisations should be consulted and involved in any changes to job descriptions, roles and responsibilities. Consideration should be given to the introduction of the NOS for Working with Parents and the Common Core of Skills and Knowledge for the Children's Workforce to ensure a competent, safe and up-to-date workforce. Public protection and safeguarding issues need to be considered.

Other factors to be examined are:

- Who has responsibility and accountability for which staff groups and work areas? In which of these areas is there potential to introduce skill mix, or are there other solutions?
- Consideration needs to be given to the safeguards and organisational structures need to be in place to ensure that skill mix provides safe, cost effective and satisfactory care.
- Where skill mix has already been introduced or is being considered, it is vital to ensure that the Nursing & Midwifery Council (NMC) registrant leading the team is given the opportunity to develop leadership and mentoring skills. Support from the employing authority will be needed to ensure that the team leader has the time to properly induct skill mix staff and that caseloads are of an appropriate size to enable this to be managed safely.

What changes need to be made in practice?

- Will it be a mix of posts?
- A change in staff deployment across the area?
- A change of roles for current staff or staff groups?
- Will you introduce new roles/staff groups?

In addition to the above Buchan and May (2000) suggest consideration needs to be given to the financial, resource, legislative and regulatory constraints which may arise from the organisational contexts. This will vary in the four different countries within the UK.

STAGE 3

This involves considering the resources available. Different approaches will require different levels and types of resources. It is important to accurately evaluate the following:

- Staff time needed.
- The skills and training that will be needed.
- The information technology resources that may be required.
- Office accommodation and equipment necessary to carry out the role.
- Geographical area to be covered, possible constraints associated with this, lone worker policy, liaison and communication protocols.
- The extra management resources required to manage a skill mix team also need to be factored in.
- Can all the direct and indirect costs be met including any training or staff redeployment?

STAGE 4

This requires a thorough exploration of the selection and implementation of the skill mix approach selected. The following questions need to be considered:

- What is the likely level of client acceptance?
- What power relationships are there between the different stakeholders and staff groups involved in the proposed skill mix introduction?
- What is the timescale for the introduction of skill mix?
- What preparatory work needs to be done?

For a more detailed explanation of this process see Buchan (1999).

STAGE 5

Following on from this model, Unite/CPHVA would advocate that a further stage would need to be added which would review and evaluate the changes made and the impact this has had on the service and service users. This should be a spiral process using the information and experiences gained from the review to:

- Revisit the original objectives.
- Evaluate the outcome indicators and criteria for success.
- Disseminate the findings to staff.

It may be necessary to return to Stage 1 and repeat the process again.

KEY POINTS

1. A pre requisite for introducing and implementing skill mix is supportive effective management who fully understand change management principles and the stress associated with change. It is essential that everyone affected by the skill mix changes are consulted and involved in the process.

2. Consideration needs to be given to the safeguards, and organisational structures need to be in place to ensure that skill mix provides safe, cost effective and satisfactory care.
3. Job roles and descriptions must be based on the needs of the service users and should be reviewed and updated regularly. Clients and families need to be involved in this process and the service evaluated in conjunction with them to determine the level of client acceptance.

Considerations for practice

Matching staff skills to meet protocol outcomes

Each employing authority will need to work with its own clinical governance group to produce protocols that are required for their population and enable each employee's skills and abilities to be fully used. The focus of any, and every protocol, must be to examine each step in the work of the team, to identify what is being delivered, its value, the level of skill required and how the work can be shared. Examining work from a Portage perspective would involve breaking a task down and analysing all the different components that make up the task. There needs to be a measure or assessment of the level of skill required to carry out a task, rather than the skill itself, as practitioners need to make visible the cognitive characteristic of the task. This is an important distinction to understand as activity analysis only examines the visible manual aspects of a task but the decision making process, professional judgement and clinical observations go undocumented. An example would be the theoretical knowledge base and experience level required to detect and safely manage domestic abuse. Assessment can often appear to be intuitive in nature and not just based on analytical principles such as those encouraged in a nursing model.

Matching models to suit the needs and skill mix of individual areas

Community staff and practitioners within the skill mix team will all have had different training and experience so it is important that previous training and knowledge is taken into account and that there is flexibility within the system. This should enable skill mix staff and teams to develop their own models to match the needs and skill mix to the individual areas in which they work. It would also allow skill mix staff to map the specific work/tasks they undertake and this could be considered in a "Portage steps" type approach to some of the work undertaken.

Before introducing skill mix it would be a useful exercise to analyse which mix and level of skills would be most beneficial for the needs of the families/patients/clients and the environment of care, they work in. Using this model, risk can be identified and then systems put in place to deliver services and support the development of skill mix staff. This may include putting specific training in place for some staff.

Recognising competence

Highly skilled professionals become unconsciously competent at the work they do which can lead them to underestimate the skills needed to perform their role. To a casual observer health visiting can appear an easy job as what you see on the outside hides the internal processes and higher cognitive skills being used. It is often only when supervising/working with other professionals, students and newly qualified staff or during supervision or reflective practice, that the tacit skills and knowledge being used become explicit and apparent. All new skills take time to acquire and for the person to become competent at using them, not unlike learning to drive a car. The process of learning and reflective practice is a continuous cycle and helps to refine and develop professional practice and skills.

All newly qualified staff, staff new in post or to working in the community, will require time to develop competency in their new role. The learning model below in Figure 6, illustrates the stages of learning individuals go through to acquire competency in new skills. The progression is from quadrant 1 through 2 and 3 to 4. It is not possible to jump stages. For some skills, especially advanced ones, people can regress to previous stages, particularly from 4 to 3, or from 3 to 2 if they fail to practice and exercise their new skills. A person regressing from 4, back through 3, to 2, will need to develop again through 3 to achieve stage 4 – unconscious competence again. For certain skills, in certain roles, Stage 3, conscious competence, is perfectly adequate. Stage 4 is when it becomes second nature, or the practitioner can teach others the skills involved at this level of practice.. This stage also gives rise to the need for long-standing unconscious competence to be checked periodically against new standards.

It has been suggested that a fifth stage in this cycle exists, reflective competence – a step beyond unconscious competence. This involves being conscious of your own unconscious competence and looking at it from the outside and trying to understand how the theories, models and beliefs inform what I do now and how I do it. These theories and beliefs may be different to the ones that were learnt consciously and then became unconscious. They may include new ones that have been learnt since and incorporated into existing knowledge and experience that can form part of a practitioner's expertise and are only found at an advanced level of practice. It indicates a stage where you can operate with fluency yourself on an instinctive level, but are also able to articulate what you are doing for yourself and others. This advanced skill in practice is rarely acknowledged, but is essential for teaching skill mix staff and mentoring and supervising staff of all grades.

All staff however experienced or senior require regular protected time for supervision with a skilled supervisor. Supervision forms an essential part of reflective practice and professional development. This should be in addition to safeguarding supervision and forms an important part of the clinical governance for all registered nurses.

In a nursing skill mix review undertaken by Newcastle Community Health by Coomber *et al* (1992), an in-depth study was made of the skills applied by nursing staff in a variety of tasks. All community staff kept diaries for a week that identified the tasks undertaken and the skills used for that task.

The vast range of skills used in the apparent simple task of telephone calls by health visitors clearly demonstrates the range of intricate interactions occurring such as decision making, negotiation, counselling and information giving all requiring a robust knowledge base. In the same task, examples given by community nursery nurses used some of the same skills, however the community nursery nurse identified

Figure 6: Competency Self-evaluation Model

Adapted from businessballs website model http://www.businessballs.com/consciouscompetencelearningmodel.htm (accessed 20th October 2008)

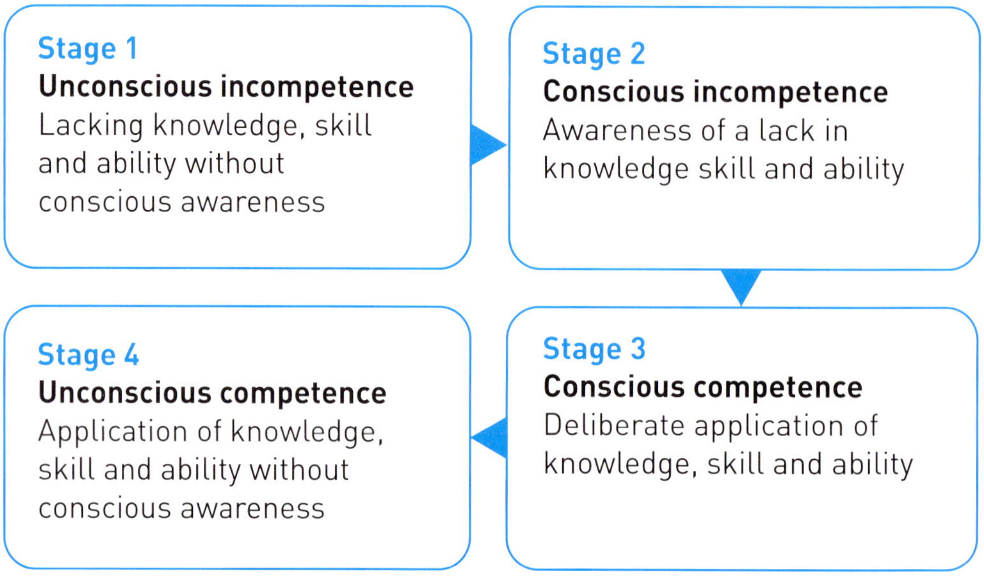

Stage 1 **Unconscious incompetence** Lacking knowledge, skill and ability without conscious awareness	Stage 2 **Conscious incompetence** Awareness of a lack in knowledge skill and ability
Stage 4 **Unconscious competence** Application of knowledge, skill and ability without conscious awareness	Stage 3 **Conscious competence** Deliberate application of knowledge, skill and ability

skills such as memory, numeracy, writing and concentration as important in this task whilst the health visitor used a much wider range of higher cognitive skills. From this same study a similar pattern can be observed when the other task are performed by health visitors and nursery nurses. Similarly, a wider variety of higher cognitive skills were used by the health visitors, including peripheral skills such as expressive, instrumental and organisational skills.

These examples highlight the internal processes and tacit knowledge and skills health visitors used when performing the same task. It also underlines the points previously made regarding the differing levels of skills required to carry out tasks and the higher cognitive processes, such as decision making, managing ambiguity, balancing risk,, analysing complex situations, using professional judgement and clinical observation that skills are invisible when the same task is performed by highly trained and experienced practitioners. As child maltreatment and domestic abuse are frequently missed or underreported, it is essential that there is a robust genetic universal service delivered by educated, skilled and experienced practitioners to protect children and vulnerable adults.

It is not possible to directly compare the skills used when conducting developmental assessments for the two different groups as this was only examined in relation to the health visitor. Developmental assessments use a complex skill network incorporating the search for health needs and facilitation of health-enhancing activities. One could hypothesise that a similar pattern may be noticeable. It is apparent from the practice examples in Chapter 3 that the more skilled professional performs the task at a much higher and more in-depth level. This is one of the complexities of managing skill mix staff and delegating work appropriately. There needs to be a measure of the skill level required to carry out a task rather than just identifying the skill itself.

It should also be noted that it is often assumed that every task can be carried out within a specific period of time, which implies that every client has the same set of circumstances and, realistically, this is rarely the case.

Reacting to changing needs in service

Anxiety regarding skill mix is often due to how it is implemented by managers when faced with changing needs or circumstances in practice. Often economics drivers and expediency i.e. using what is available and not planning in a proactive way to employ specific skills can be the precursor for an inappropriate skill mix formula in teams. Serious concerns have been expressed regarding the community nursery nurse carrying out family health needs assessments because their training does not equip them to conduct health needs assessments and see the interactions between health conditions, medications and the language of illness.

The *Community Nursery Nurse Professional Guidelines* produced by Unite/CPHVA (2007), give very clear guidance (page3 that community nursery nurses should not be undertaking clinical and public health assessments.

Equally consideration needs to be given to an unintended change of service when different personnel are used. For example, school nurses previously offered health assessments to all five year olds. Now, many PCTs and employing authorities have delegated the tasks of checking height, weight, vision and hearing to a health care assistant or nursery nurse, which results in a different outcome. When a qualified school nurse carries out a health assessment, they use all their knowledge and expertise of child development, combined with information from the teacher, the health visitor and the parent; to assess the child's health needs. This holistic assessment ensures that any problems are identified and treatment or referral offered. School nurses' higher level skills allow them to pick out vulnerable children and ensure that they have access to services, are followed up, and liaise with other professionals as necessary.

Safeguarding children – a public health priority

A crucial part of any skill mix implementation plan needs to consider public protection and safeguarding children and vulnerable adults.

> In the recently published biennial analysis of serious case reviews 2003–2005, one of the key findings from this research report by Brandon *et al* (2008) was that ⅔ of the 161 children studied died and a ⅓ were seriously injured. **47 % of these were children under 1 and only 12% of the 161 children were on the child protection register.** This emphasises the necessity of a robust health visiting service delivered by highly trained, skilled professionals who are alert to the ways in which difficulties and protective factors interact if they are to understand the infant/child's experience and how significant harm might arise. The review highlighted the fact that less qualified staff did not challenge families, rather accepted what they were told.

Introducing skill mix

It is worth considering some of the key messages from Brandon et al's report (2008) and the implications these may have for employing authorities, commissioners of services, managers, community practitioners and other skill mix staff in maintaining adequate, safe services to protect children and families. The population paradox described below also indicates why a population approach to prevention and detection of child maltreatment is essential.

1. If management structures and staff support systems collapse due to an excessive workload, the result is often paralysis in the workers, or ill health, or absenteeism or other signs of stress. The *NHS Staff Survey* conducted by the Healthcare Commission (2006) revealed that 45 % of health visitors in PCTs were suffering from work-related stress.
2. Good support is needed so that practitioners can work effectively with complex cases. Practitioners must be self-aware, flexible and sensitive to the factors underlying their own and the family's behaviour and emotions.
3. Supervision helps practitioners to think, to explain and to understand. It also helps them to cope with the complex emotional demands of work with children and their families. Adequate protected time for safeguarding supervision is essential.
4. Most serious child abuse is essentially unpredictable – even if the "whole picture" had been known, it would not have been possible to anticipate serious abuse for most of the children at the centre of the reviews highlighted above. This emphasises the risk of providing a very selective service to families who are deemed to be "vulnerable" (Rose, 1993). A robust universal service is essential for safeguarding and public protection (see the population paradox below for further exploration of this).
5. There were numerous childhood adversities (including indicators of recurrence of maltreatment), in the majority of the cases but these were not known to all of the professionals involved prior to the serious case review being undertaken. There are serious professional concerns that the lack of a personalised service from a named health visitor is now resulting in more children being missed.
6. It is crucial for professionals to feel that they, and their employing agency, have done their best for the child. Some health visitors feel that they are unable to offer the support and services that such families require due to staffing issues and lack of resources (Adams & Craig, 2007, 2008). This may lead to an increase in work-related stress (Healthcare Commission, 2008).
7. Early detection of parenting difficulties is crucial so that timely help can be offered. This early detection is dependent on building up trusting, therapeutic relationships with families which requires time for families to develop trust in the practitioner.
8. "Hard to reach" families need flexible, individually-tailored services.
9. Early intervention and working with early needs is part of the safeguarding continuum and not a separate sphere of activity.
10. The families of very young children who were physically assaulted tended to have the least, or the briefest contact with children's social care which puts a greater onus on universal agencies to recognise signs of harm to children, again highlighting the importance of health visitors conducting these initial assessments.
11. All practitioners need a holistic understanding of children and families and need training about the way in which separate factors might interact to cause increased stresses in the family and increased risks of harm to the child.

Health visitors, school nurses and all practitioners who have contact with children and families need to be mindful of these messages from research and the implications for practice and skill mix staff. Practitioners are encouraged to bring this information to the attention of managers and commissioners of services, to ensure that the services provided for children and families adequately safeguard them.

The population paradox

The above biennial analysis of serious case reviews 2003–2005 (Brandon *et al*, 2008), and key findings particularly points four, five, nine, 10 and 11, support Rose's (1993) and Barlow and Stewart Brown's (2003) argument that the bulk of problems in society arise in the many who are not necessarily high risk rather than the few who are high risk. The reason for this is that there are a very large number who are not at especially high risk.

Child abuse, domestic abuse and depression are common problems that health visitors deal with regularly. To detect and prevent child maltreatment a population level approach is essential (Barlow and Stewart Brown, 2003). For this to be effective practitioners need time to develop trusting relationship with families and conduct holistic assessments which are a process and not a one-off assessment completed in a single visit. This finding is a recurrent theme throughout this book. Despite this repeated thesis in the literature and research, it is a factor not always understood and appreciated by commissioners and managers of services. The focus often appears to be on the tasks to be performed, rather than appreciating the skill level required to conduct holistic family needs health assessments. The danger with targeting services at those of high risk is that there is a danger of leaving untouched vast swathes of those with health and social problems. Rose (1993), states that no screening instrument can be sufficiently precise to accurately identify those most likely to suffer problems. This can make delegation of duties in skill mix teams more complex as it is often difficult to make accurate assessments unless you have developed good relationships with your families. This requires time a commodity often in short supply in many health visiting teams today, as the research by Cowley *et al* (2007) indicates and as reported by Adams and Craig (2007 and 2008).

KEY POINTS

Factors for successful skill mix introduction:

- A "bottom-up" approach.
- Excellent leadership.
- Clear lines of communication and accountability.
- Clearly thought-through planning and implementation.
- Regular planned supervision.
- Thorough induction training and programme for all new staff.
- Clear and established links with clinical governance to produce protocols.
- Regular appraisal and training to ensure professional development.
- Maintenance of core competencies.
- Adequate resources for the team.
- Regular review of the skill mix team with team members.
- Clear objectives and outcomes for each team member that are audited regularly.

Conclusion

As this book has demonstrated it is important for community practitioners, their managers and commissioners of services to have a clear understanding of the essential differences between grade mix/skill substitution and skill mix. Furthermore, to understand the implications of the team makeup for effective and efficient practice, and the delivery of quality and productive services.

It is clear that the amount of time needed to implement and manage skill mix teams is frequently underestimated. It is hence imperative that dedicated time and authority is given to the lead practitioners so they can ensure their teams operate effectively and safely. Ultimately, the success of any team will be dependent on the leadership and planning that underpins its constitution and activity.

Research has not kept pace with the changes in community practice and there is regrettably limited knowledge on substitution activity and safe working practices of different practitioners, and support workers, in a skill mix team. This needs to be rectified urgently. For skill mix to be fully accepted by staff, evidence is required that, when appropriately constituted, the advantages of the chosen team skill mix to client outcomes, outweighs any disadvantages.

Despite the limited nature of the evidence base for skill mix in the community setting, lessons can be drawn from studies in acute and other settings. It is therefore important that managers contemplating introducing, or revising, a skill mix team consider carefully the key issues discussed in this book in order to get it right from the start. The whole thrust of the recent policy initiatives led by Lord Darzi and the Transforming Community Services series, Ambition, Action Achievement, for community health activity in England, is to put the control back with the clinicians, reinstating them as service leaders so they must be a key part of any discussions.

A thorough understanding is required of the complexity of delegation in community settings. The lines of accountability and delegation dilemmas staff may be exposed to, need to be fully appreciated by practitioners, managers and the commissioners of services. NMC registrants, whether managers or practitioners, must be clear on their duty of care and what is acceptable delegation, or they could risk facing a professional misconduct hearing.

McKenna's (1995) work clearly demonstrates how a rich mix of mainly qualified staff may enhance service quality as against using more unqualified staff. Getting the mix wrong has knock on effects such as staff shortages through sickness and low morale, as well as affecting the quality of the service delivered. It is important that community practitioners have an understanding of such dynamics and use it to lobby for appropriately constituted skill mix teams.

Parental/client expectation and entitlement to service quality is another important issue to consider in the skill mix debate. The NHS Constitution (2009) clearly sets out, for the first time, a patient's/client's legal right to access quality services provided by appropriately qualified and experienced staff.

A final thought...

> *"Quality is difficult to measure and most of the important effects of qualified staff are invisible to the naked eye".* (McKenna, 1995, p457)

Recommendations

Recommendation 1

Skill mix decisions are based on determining the combination of skills necessary to deliver safe, high quality care and achieve the desired outcomes for clients, not on staff substitution on economic grounds.

Recommendation 2

The government urgently invests in research:

- To evaluate the outcomes for children and families with well funded universal provision in pre-school and school health services.
- To determine the public health cost/benefits of various models of skill mix in community nursing teams.
- To explore the effects of models of skill mix on staff stress, client satisfaction and staff turnover.
- To ascertain whether delegation of health visitor tasks to other health care team members, affects the outcomes of "soft" areas of care such as health promotion or psychological support.
- To determine the outcomes for families in relation to domestic violence, postnatal depression and safeguarding children of health visitors working in skill mixed teams as opposed to delivering solely health visitor interventions in these instances.
- To identify which models of intervention can be used, and by whom, to achieve the best outcomes for children and families.

Recommendation 3

Development and standardisation of national core competencies for community staff nurses, community nursery nurses, community health care assistants, support workers working in health visiting, school nursing or district nursing teams.

Recommendation 4

Development and standardisation of national induction training for community staff so they can be adequately prepared for the job they will be required to do.

Recommendation 5

That the Care Quality Commission monitors skill mix decisions as part of their safeguarding reviews.

Recommendation 6

Guidance from the Department of Health and the NMC on minimum and maximum numbers of children specialist community public health nurses can be professionally accountable for. In areas of high deprivation and areas where there are many vulnerable children, these numbers need to be reduced very significantly to ensure health gain.

Recommendation 7

The government issues clear guidance on safe skill mix ratios in community practice, for health visiting and school nursing teams. This needs to reflect the health needs of the local community.

Frequently asked questions (FAQs)

What is the employer's responsibility with regard to work induced stress and skill mix working arrangements?

The employing authority has a duty of care to its staff as illustrated in the following case study where a health visitor successfully sued the employer after suffering a psychiatric breakdown induced by work-related stress.

> A health visitor started work for a new Primary Care Trust in 2000 working 28 hours/week. On starting, she was told that her caseload would not exceed 200. By 2002, this had increased to 230–240. Due to increased levels of sickness and absence in the trust, the work demands increased until, after several meetings with her line manager, the health visitor needed to go off sick. The health visitor was unable to return to work in that role due to stress and took a more junior post resulting in a drop of £9,000 a year in salary. In court she received over £61,000 in damages.
>
> Full text can be viewed at: *http://www.casetrack.com/ct4plc.nsf/items/6-214-1000* (Also reported in *Community Practitioner,* Feb. 2007).

The *NHS Staff Survey* (2008) conducted by the Healthcare Commission revealed that 41% of health visitors (38% of community nurses) in PCTs were suffering from work-related stress. http://www.healthcarecommission.org.uk/nationalfindings/surveys/healthcareprofessionals/surveysofnhsstaff/2006.cfm

Comment: It is possible to suggest there may be a link between the increase in work-related stress and the concurrent decrease in the numbers of health visitors. This, coupled with the spread of corporate working models introduced in many areas to compensate for the decrease in WTE health visitors, and the corresponding rise in caseload numbers, and the introduction of more grade mix staff. Add to this the additional management, supervision and training of skill mix staff and it is not difficult to begin to understand some of the underlying reasons behind the increase in work-related stress for SCPHNs.

The costs of stress not only affect the individual concerned, but affect the whole service in terms of the investigation costs and time, the cost of the payout and the effects it has on other staff who have to cover long-term sick leave. This, is turn, impacts on the service provided to patients/families and the outcomes for children.

Work-induced stress is widely recognised as a significant problem in the NHS. The Health and Safety Executive (HSE) recognises that workers in health and social care have some of the highest rates of self-reported illness due to stress and anxiety. The

HSE reports that stress, anxiety and depression accounts for an estimated 12.8 million self-reported working days lost each year. Thirty per cent of sickness absence in the NHS is due to stress and costs £300-£400 million per year. Stress also contributes to accidents and errors by employers, low morale and poor performance (see the Low Morale Cycle, McKenna (1995), on page 21 for an illustration of this); consequently, the NHS cannot afford to ignore work-related stress.

The NHS has a legal obligation to prevent or reduce work-associated stress. In 2001 the HSE published guidance on *Tackling Work-related Stress: a Manager's Guide to Improving and Maintaining Employee Health and Well Being* (HSG, 218). This guidance highlights the major role managers can play in reducing the problems of stress and how to take a proactive approach in this.

The HSE has now issued management standards of good practice that employers can use to measure their manager's performance in tackling a range of key stressors. One NHS trust has been issued with a compliance notice for failing to carry out assessments of the risks to staff or work-related stress. See http://www.hse.gov.uk/stress/index.htm

Excessive workload and responsibility need to be addressed, and taken seriously. The increasing use of grade/skill mix in primary healthcare teams and the additional delegating responsibility and accountability this entails, can cause serious stress and ill health. It is vital that the requisite supportive management and supervision necessary to support staff is available, and that the practitioners' concerns are listened to, and taken seriously. A management culture that is sympathetic to staff suffering from occupational stress, and is prepared to act to alleviate it, can make a real difference to the outcome.

What is the health visitor's role in skill mix teams?

Within skill mix teams health visitors are both leaders and expert practitioners. The recent *Review of Health Visiting* (DH, 2007), recognised health visitors as highly trained professionals who should be *"responsible for the 'difficult things'",* these were identified as the following:

- Managing risk/decision making in conditions of uncertainty, including safeguarding children.
- Building therapeutic relationships and addressing difficult issues in families with complex needs.
- Leading multi-skilled teams.
- Working across sectors and putting health into multi-agency work.
- Delivering population level outcomes.
- Assessment and identification of existing and future vulnerability.
- Engaging hard to reach groups and individuals.
- Translating evidence into practice.
(Facing the Future, DH, 2007, p7)

Comment: Whilst welcoming the recognition of the skills of health visitors, professional concern has been expressed that the proposed skill mix increases, and

Frequently asked questions (FAQs)

the targeting of health visitors to work with conspicuous need and vulnerable families, will make early identification and intervention impossible. The health visiting review appears to be being interpreted, in some PCTs, as that health visitors should only work with vulnerable families and those with complex needs, this is leading to the subsequent withdrawal of health visitors from universal home visiting. The serious consequences arising from this are reported in the 14th annual Unite/CPHVA *Omnibus Survey 2008,* by Adams and Craig (2008).

Building therapeutic relationships lies at the heart of community practice, and is integral to all the work the health visitor undertakes. This relationship provides the context and, is the vehicle for, the work community practitioners do in partnership with parents. Branson, Badger and Dodds (2003), have expressed concern that skill mix may affect the building of therapeutic relationships. In Unite/CPHVA's *Response to Facing the Future* (Unite/CPHVA, 2007), anxiety was expressed by CPHVA members that there was insufficient understanding of the time needed to develop relationships with clients. Many members described the negative impact the reduction in the workforce, and training budgets, was having on the ability of health visitors to maintain standards and provide a satisfactory health visiting service. Members also reported that there appeared to be a lack of understanding of the breadth and purpose of health visiting in some areas at local, regional and strategic level. This was further reinforced by the often large gap between local implementation and the national policy.

An important issue is the supervision the health visitor is able to give in a skill mix team in terms of safeguarding issues. Health visitors are often working part-time, and manage heavy, intense caseloads as well as supervising junior grade staff. What time/experience/training do they have for effective supervision of the team generally and in terms of specific child protection supervision? It has been suggested, by experienced safeguarding practitioners, that a lot of important information is never discussed because of lack of time. A very important aspect of safeguarding is prevention and the skilled holistic health needs assessment by the health visitor is required to identify early parenting difficulties, and effective early intervention, before there is significant harm.

What constitutes skill mix in health visiting teams?

Skill mix in health visiting is not only about community staff nurses or community nursery nurses; skill mix may be much wider including community health educators, health care assistants, interpreters, volunteers and administrative support. Volunteers such as community mothers, Home Start workers, and breastfeeding peer supporters may all form part of the skill mix staff. All of these roles are part of a children's service that parents may choose to use. There is a difference between skill mix in traditional primary health care teams and Sure Start skill mix teams led by health visitors. The Sure Start model has access to a much wider pool of multi-disciplinary skills (such as primary mental health workers, social workers, community psychiatric nurses, midwives, psychologists, play therapists, portage workers, interpreters, dieticians, debt counsellors etc), rather than the usual family of nursing skill mix found in many primary health care teams. In all models of service delivery, if parents, carers and children are to use the service effectively, they need to understand how to access it, and the different roles within the team.

Many health visitors are now working corporately. In 2008 Adams and Craig reported that over 62% of health visitors had a corporate caseload. The evidence from the 2008 Omnibus Survey (Adams and Craig), also seemed to suggest that corporate working has been used as a method of reducing health visitor numbers, whilst trying to manage the resultant risk to vulnerable children, as those working corporately had significantly higher caseloads. This is of concern as 69.2% of health visitors also said that they no longer had the resources to respond to the needs of the most vulnerable children on their caseloads. Furthermore, they were unable to deliver the required evidence-based inputs in line with the Public Service Agreement targets (PSA), to protect the health of children and tackle health inequalities. Twenty-five per cent of health visitors from this survey said they feared another child death, such as Victoria Climbié, where they worked. This is a major concern, and subsequent high profile child abuse deaths such as the 17-month-old toddler, Baby Peter, reinforce the seriousness of this professional alarm.

National job profiles for health visitors, specialist health visitors and health visiting specialist community practice teachers are available at: http://www.nhsemployers.org/PayAndContracts/AgendaForChange/NationalJobProfiles/Pages/NursingAndMidwifery.aspx

What questions and issues need to be considered *BEFORE* skill mix is introduced?

Below are some questions that may be useful for practitioners, managers, or teams to consider before introducing skill mix or if they are reviewing existing skill mix provision.

- Are we introducing skill mix or grade mix (see pages 6–7) for a definition and discussion of this? Skill mix and grade mix are very different and it is important to be clear about the differences between them.
- What safeguards and organisational structures need to be implemented to ensure that skill/grade mix provides safe, cost effective and satisfactory care?
- What changes to the training of Specialist Community Public Health Nurses (SCPHN) and skill mix staff, will be necessary in future to ensure that the potential benefits of skill mix are realised?
- What changes in the induction programme and professional development training will be needed to prepare and equip staff for working in skill/grade mix teams?
- Under what circumstances can some activities be safely delegated to a team member who is not a health visitor or school nurse?
- Will the problem to be solved be addressed by introducing skill/grade mix changes? Is this the best solution? There may be other more appropriate methods for dealing with the problems.
- Is the use of skill/grade mix to solve problems of the short supply of health visitors and qualified school nurses, simply moving the problem of shortages further down the professional chain?

Frequently asked questions (FAQs)

- Where skill/grade mix has already been introduced, or is being considered, it is vital to ensure that the Nursing & Midwifery Council (NMC) registrant leading the team is given the opportunity to develop leadership and mentoring skills. Support from the employing authority will be needed to ensure that the team leader has the time to properly induct skill/grade mix staff and that caseloads are of an appropriate size to enable this to be managed safely.

What questions and issues need to be considered *AFTER* skill mix is introduced?

- Do clients and families find the service provided using skill/grade mix models as satisfactory as those provided by traditional models?
- Has the workload of highly trained professionals increased in practice by the use of skill/grade mix? The increased supervision, training and management of the skill/grade mix team and the need to provide increasing numbers of protocols to ensure safe practice and quality of care needs to be taken into consideration.
- Review and evaluate the changes made and the impact this has had on the service, service users and partner agencies.
- Is the induction programme and training provided sufficient to prepare staff for working in skill/grade mix teams?

Why does a Family Health Needs Assessment need to be done by a health visitor?

The aim of the Family Health Needs Assessment (FHNA) is to undertake a full assessment of the family's health and parenting needs. In particular, the impact of parenting capacity and family and environmental factors on the child's health and well being must be explored and those families who may require additional support identified. A family health plan will be developed from this as appropriate, in partnership with family members. This assessment should also be used as an opportunity to identify positive factors and strengths.

The training that health visitors and school nurses receive enables them to understand the bio-medical model of health and its importance in disease aetiology (pathogenesis) but their practice is developed from their primary interest in what creates health (salutogenesis) (Cowley and Frost, 2006). This is one aspect that sets health visiting and school nursing apart from traditional nursing.

The breadth and depth of the health visitor's knowledge in these areas, together with her/his expert skills in health needs assessment, enables her/him to search for health needs at an individual, family and population level. The health visitor is then able to coordinate the work of the team according to these identified needs. This is important to acknowledge as this skilled family health needs assessment needs to be carried out on every family to identify who may require extra support or intensive visiting.

How can the skills of community staff nurses (CSN) best be used to enhance the health visiting service?

Staff nurses are registered nurses, some come with a wide range of skill and experience; others are relatively less experienced. All can contribute a range of input to a children service's team, 0–18 years, not just 0–5.

Professionally, they have to act in accordance with the NMC *Code of Professional Conduct* (2008), with particular reference to acknowledge the strengths and limitations of their competence in order to safeguard the well being of patients, carers and clients.

Key issues and questions when employing staff nurses to work with health visitors are:

1. **Recruitment and selection:** Should only nurses who are trained to work with children and families be considered? When recruiting, can this post be seen as a route into health visiting for the staff nurse and are the appropriate training and development opportunities in place?
2. **Induction:** Who is responsible, and for how long, what are the induction procedures in the differing trusts or employing authorities?
3. **Training of staff nurses:** All are trained nurses and, as such, are competent to understand and discuss health issues and give immunisations. They are trained in areas of awareness of the needs of vulnerable adults/children but not all will have had formal community training. Some employing authorities offer community training modules at local universities and other higher education institutes alongside community practice tutors providing local training. Others have local protocols and competency-based tasks that are monitored and signed off. Some have local "on the job training" that may have less structure. This issue needs considerable debate and exploration. It is intrinsically linked to the competence development of all staff in children's services.
4. **Risk assessment:** Tasks and delegated duties need to be assessed from a risk assessment viewpoint to ensure safe standards of practice. What is in place to ensure that the staff nurses are working to a required standard, and is it clear who is responsible for monitoring them? Some areas have developed core competencies for community staff nurses based on the KSF dimensions. See also Unite/CPHVA publications.

The tasks most frequently undertaken by community staff nurses in health visiting skill mix teams are:

- Selected transfer in visits.
- Accident and emergency follow up.
- Home safety/prevention of accidents advice.
- Specific follow up visits.
- Immunisations.
- Clinic support.
- Health promotion.
- Supporting families who have children with disabilities.
- Specific home visits for children with disabilities i.e. continence reassessment.

Frequently asked questions (FAQs)

- Childhood illness and ailments.
- Infant feeding, weaning information/support, diet and healthy family nutrition and support.
- Group work with the health visitor.
- Breastfeeding support and baby massage.
- Follow up of non attendance for appointments.
- Working with the school health service.
- Smoking cessation intervention/support.
- Alcohol use.
- Sexual health/family planning.
- Activity and exercise.
- Public health activities.

5. **Monitoring and development of skill mix:** It is most likely that the health visitor or team leader will have responsibility for monitoring standards and competencies within the team, as well as considering the training and development needs of the members and the team as a whole. This raises issues around whether all health visitors are competent or adequately trained to take on this additional role.

Any community staff nurse development plan should be flexible and delivered over a timescale that is realistic and in keeping with the workload demands and client needs. The precise content of the development plan will be determined by, and be in keeping with, the skills and competencies that the individual staff nurse brings and the skills requirements of the health visitor team and client group. The development process should be supported by reflection and an on-going assessment of individual learning needs, and the team development plan.

The staff nurse skill mix role within the health visiting service could support the skills escalator approach to developing the workforce. It can provide the opportunity for widening access to the specialist practitioner programme and support both capability building and increasing the capacity of health visitor service delivery if skill mix is used appropriately.

A variety of assessment methods could be used, such as:

- Discussion with mentor.
- Questions and answers – health visitor mentor and nurse.
- Observation in the workplace.
- Self-assessment.
- Clinical supervision.
- Reflective practice and maintenance of a reflective log.
- Peer review.

Examples of a community staff nurse national profile is available at: http://www.nhsemployers.org/PayAndContracts/AgendaForChange/NationalJobProfiles/Documents/Community_services.pdf

How can the skill of community nursery nurses (CNN) best be used to enhance the health visiting service?

The community nursery nurse is an important professional within a community nursing/health visiting team and children's services. They have specific child focused expertise but are not registered nurses. They are able to undertake delegated activities associated with children of 0–8 years of age. These activities should be provided through shared packages of care. Community nursery nurses may also work with young people aged eight to 19 years, and adults, providing them with health promotion initiatives and advice.

Any nursery nurse who is working in the community or primary care should have attained one of the following qualifications:

- NNEB, now replaced by the Diploma in Childcare and Education (DCE) awarded by CACHE and the HNC in Child Care and Education (Scotland)

- Level 3 BTEC National Diploma in Early Years, awarded by EDEXCEL.

- NVQ/SNVQ Level 3 in Early Years and Education, awarded by City & Guilds, CACHE, EDEXCEL and the OU.

The Qualification and Curriculum Authority (QCA) recommends the above qualifications over any other qualifications, as they have the necessary theoretical and practical training in child development.

Community nursery nurses may train and be competent in aspects of parenting and health promotion that will equip them to work with parents and young people to enable these clients to enhance their health and that of the family unit. Community nursery nurses may train in leadership, mentorship and as an assessor to enable them to lead other community nursery nurses.

Community nursery nurses should never be accountable for a caseload. They cannot replace the clinical and public health assessments that health visitors and other NMC registrants perform. Community nursery nurses should *not* undertake the following:

- New birth visits.
- Unknown transfers in (not living previously within the health visiting teams locality).
- Postnatal depression assessments and initial listening visits.
- Known challenging families – they should not visit alone, nor should any other staff member be placed in a risky situation. (All PCTs and employing authorities will have lone worker policies).
- Caseload responsibilities.

Community nursery nurses need a competency framework that covers all aspects of their work (see Unite/CPHVA's *Competency Framework and Best Practice Guidelines*, Oct. 2006).

Frequently asked questions (FAQs)

Clerical duties are best undertaken by an appropriately trained person as part of the team. It is not the best use of resources to use community nursery nurses, NMC registrants or other clinical professionals to undertake these activities.

Community nursery nurses need appropriate leadership, managerial support and clinical supervision. Time needs to be set aside to establish good professional working relationships, to develop an understanding of what expertise and skills other skill/grade mix staff have, and what skills gaps there are.

The *Community Nursery Nurse Professional Guidance* (2007), suggests that there are a number of essential training sessions that a community nursery nurse will need to attend. See also Unite/CPHVA: *Recommended Induction Programme* for a *Community Nursery Nurse* (2007) for more detail, and a comprehensive training programme.

Training needs to be provided within the employing organisation, but will normally include:

- Fire Safety.
- Health and Safety.
- Moving and handling.
- Basic life support.
- Safeguarding children.
- Equal opportunities, equality and diversity.
- Risk management and clinical governance.
- Record keeping.
- Confidentiality, consent and data protection (Caldicott policy and information sharing guidance).
- Lone working.

All community nursery nurses must undertake training in consent during their induction and at all times follow the local policies and procedures. There are a number of areas for professional development that can enhance team working and improve client care. A community nursery nurse through his/her PDR, and/or PDP, may wish to access courses to enhance awareness in such areas as:

- Public health.
- Health promotion.
- Infant child and nutrition.
- Child and maternal mental health.
- Child and adult abuse.
- Managing groups.
- Parenting support.
- Crèche work.
- Computer skills.
- Growth monitoring.
- Reflective practice.

The NMC *Professional Code of Conduct* (2008), states very clearly an NMC registrant's responsibility when delegating work and aspects of care to others:

> *"You must establish that anyone you delegate to is able to carry out your instructions".*
>
> *"You must confirm that the outcome of any delegated task meets required standards".*
>
> *"You must make sure that everyone you are responsible for is supervised and supported".*
>
> (NMC, The Code, 2008, p6)

When delegating work, the health visitor or school nurse should document exactly what is expected of the community nursery nurse and the plans for reviewing the care plan. It is good practice for this to be in the client's record and may also include a referral form and plan with review periods documented (*Record Keeping & the Law*, Newland, 2007 and see the NMC *Advice on Delegation for Registered Nurses and Midwives,* 2008).

The delegating registrant needs to ensure that adequate supervision, support and follow up are provided.

Examples of skill mix work often undertaken by nursery nurses, is provided below. This will vary in different areas depending on local need and the skills, competence, knowledge and experience of the community nursery nurse.

- Helping at child health/school health clinics.
- Helping run parents support groups with other team members.
- Baby massage.
- Breastfeeding information and support.
- Weaning information/support.
- Infant feeding and food management.
- Child health and development assessments on children up to eight years of age.
- Smoking cessation advice.
- Health promotion.
- Safety and accident prevention.
- Promotion of positive mental health and well being in children.
- Promoting play opportunities and working with parents on play and stimulation of their children.
- Specific follow up visits delegated by the health visitor.
- Group work with the health visitor.

When delegating child health and development assessment to community nursery nurses, consideration must be given to *Health for All Children* (Hall & Elliman, 2003) which states that:

> *"Child health professionals should have the skills to elicit and interpret an account of a child's development".* (p268)

It is essential that health visitors undertake a full family and child health assessment and developmental assessment when the child first enters the caseload. Community

Frequently asked questions (FAQs)

nursery nurses are then in a position, through delegation from the health visitor, to undertake any further child developmental assessments and refer back to the health visitor should there be any concerns.

Examples of a community nursery nurse job profile is available at: http://www.nhsemployers.org/PayAndContracts/AgendaForChange/NationalJobProfiles/Documents/Community_services.pdf

How can the skills of the community support worker (CSW) best be used to enhance the health visiting or community nursing service?

This is a really essential role within a health visiting service. The community support worker can take responsibility for ensuring the office runs smoothly by organising and monitoring the record management system and carrying out many of the routine administrative/secretarial tasks. Without an administrative assistant this work would have to be carried out by the clinical staff. As illustrated in the research by Cowley *et al* (2007), adequate administrative support was directly correlated to the provision of a more comprehensive core health visiting service.

The work that can be appropriately carried out by such a team member includes:

- Maintaining the "Central Birth Book" or other record system that is in place to determine who is on the caseload.
- Managing the record filing system so that it is easy for all staff to use.
- Filing correspondence within individual records once it has been read or actioned by the accountable NMC practitioner.
- Typing letters/referrals/reports.
- Writing up/filing carbon copies of clinic attendances by clients at clinics.
- Arranging clinics and sending out appointments.
- "Pulling" and re-filing records for pre-arranged clinics or visits.
- Supporting specialist services provided by the service, for example, by maintaining databases for the Care of the Next Infant (CONI) programme or groups or other services run by the health visiting service.
- Maintaining (including ordering) stock levels of health promotion materials and office stationery.
- Making up packs to be used at standard client contacts i.e. local information to be given at a primary visit or materials for health promotion sessions or clinic or groups.
- Taking, typing and distributing minutes of meetings.
- Answering the phone and taking messages, giving information that is requested, if it is of a straightforward, factual nature.
- Photocopying.
- Maintaining databases for the health visiting team and downloading information from the computer re referrals, new births and other important information and messages.
- Entering information on the IT system re number of contacts and other factual information required for auditing the service.

There may be a support role that includes direct client contact but this is different to the administrative role as suggested above.

The exact role requirements should be determined before the role is recruited into. If it is essential for the postholder to have touch typing, and record management skills, this should be clearly stated in the job description. If it is expected that the individual will obtain skills once employed i.e. minute taking skills, this should also be stated and the opportunity to obtain these skills once employed provided.

The higher the level of competence for the role the higher the band is likely to be. However, the increased productivity of the clinical team members who will no longer be routinely carrying out purely administrative tasks, should partly offset this increased cost (Coomber *et al*, 1992; Carr and Pearson's, 2005; Cowley *et al*, 2007; RCN, BBC News, 27th April 2008).

An example is given in Chapter 1, page 17, of how community support workers were used in more clinical roles to support health visiting teams in Glasgow to pilot a skill mix model for health visiting in the Starting Well Project (MacKenzie, 2006).

The National Job Profiles for the differing grades of clerical support workers are available at: http://www.nhsemployers.org/PayAndContracts/AgendaForChange/NationalJobProfiles/Documents/Community_services.pdf

How can the skills of volunteers best be used to enhance the health visiting and other community nursing services?

Organisations with vulnerable clients have an enhanced duty of care and they should have clear child/vulnerable adult protection policies in place. These should be reflected throughout volunteer involvement. Typical measurers might include:

- Taking up references.
- Thorough training and induction.
- Looking at working practices and making sure that all has been done to avoid unnecessary risk – for example are there ways to avoid one-to-one contact with clients?
- Adequate supervision.
- Having proper channels for clients, volunteers and staff to raise concerns.
- Actively seeking feedback from clients.

Health and Safety: Organisations have a duty of care towards their volunteers, which means, in practice, they must take all reasonable steps to avoid harm coming to them, either through their action or inaction (Section 3 of the Health & Safety at Work etc Act, 1974). (http://www.hse.gov.uk/legislation/hswa.htm).

This also places a duty on the employer *"to ensure, as far as reasonably practical, that persons not in their employment, who may be affected by their undertaking, are not exposed to risks to their health and safety"*.

Examples of the use of volunteers in community practice are community mothers, Home Start workers, breastfeeding peer supporters and interpreters.

Frequently asked questions (FAQs)

The NMC (2008), has provided an advice sheet on *Advice on Delegation for Registered Nurses and Midwives*.

The NMC code, the *Professional Code of Conduct* (2008) states:

> "You must establish that anyone you delegate to is able to carry out your instructions".
>
> "You must confirm that the outcome of any delegated task meets required standards".
>
> "You must make sure that everyone you are responsible for is supervised and supported". (NMC, The Code, 2008, p6)

Hawkins and Restall (2006), provide useful advice that needs to be borne in mind when using volunteers.

> "Volunteers can be seen as workers in the eyes of the law if they can demonstrate that they are working under a contract. A contract is a description of a relationship and is not necessarily a written document. Care should be taken to avoid creating circumstances that imply an employment relationship. In the area of employment contracts may arise where there is 'consideration' – the exchange or promise of something of material value – in return for work e.g. any money over out of pocket expenses, or a perk with a financial value e.g. training that is not necessary for the volunteer's role i.e. offering training as a benefit to the volunteer simply to improve their employment prospects". (Hawkins and Restall, 2006)

An intercollegiate information paper has been developed by the Royal College of Nursing and other professional organisations on *Supervision, Accountability and Delegation of Activities to Support Workers* (2006), which is a guide for registered practitioners and support workers that all staff need to be familiar with.

Useful links for further information about volunteers:
http://www.thecompact.org.uk
http://www.unitetheunion.com/sectors/health_sector/health_b4_profit_campaign.aspx Unite the Union, Community and not for profit sector.

What are the specific roles within school nursing skill mix teams?

The Welsh and English governments are committed to having one full-time qualified school nurse per secondary school, and its cluster of primaries, as a minimum, according to health needs. They recognise that only specialist public health nurses will deliver the change in outcomes to make the difference. Various models of working are being considered by all four countries of the UK, as it is acknowledged that there needs to be local flexibility.

In some places, health visiting and school nursing teams are working corporately as a 0–16 or 0–19 service. In Scotland, a model incorporating district nursing as well as health visiting and school nursing, has been promoted. While this offers obvious advantages to employers, it would not give an optimum service to children and young people, as inevitably, clinical need takes priority over preventative work. Schools prefer the "named nurse" role, as this is the model used by other peripatetic services and they sometimes find it harder to deal with several individuals.

As children grow into adults they want to take on responsibility for their own health choices. Consequently, a family support service such as health visiting, which is required by parents with babies, is a model which is not wanted by adolescents, who frequently want to access their own support and healthcare without the knowledge of their family.

Mental and emotional health concerns, especially bullying, stress, self-harm and risk-taking behaviour, are well documented issues in the school-aged population, leading some school nurse teams to employ CAMHS trained nurses, particularly where there are large secondary schools.

Many children and young people, who would have attended special schools in previous years, now attend mainstream school. This has posed a challenge to school staff and so community children's nurses with specialist knowledge of disabilities might work across mainstream and special schools.

In other areas school nurses are also family planning trained nurses who undertake sessional work in after school clinics and on school premises during term time, and work in well woman clinics during school holidays. They are able to do Chlamydia screening and prescribe contraception, as well as advise and educate young people, and refer if necessary.

One clinical area which is often part of the school nurses' remit is running enuresis clinics. Many of these are run by community staff nurses who have developed this as a specialism, and who may have come into school nursing via the continence service.

Some community staff nurses specialise in public health work such as reducing levels of childhood obesity using proprietary packages, or running smoking cessation groups with young people (including the issuing of nicotine patches using a patient group directive).

In view of the increasing workload, some areas now have a designated immunisation service which delivers all immunisations to school aged children. These nurses may be part of the skill mix team, or they may be managed by the public health department of the PCT or employing authority. There has been pressure from managers to employ health care assistants in this role, but this is not supported by the school nurses' professional bodies, as the qualified nurse in charge would still be professionally accountable if anything went wrong.

There are plenty of examples of joint appointments between health and education or health and children's/social services. For example, a nurse or health care worker could

Frequently asked questions (FAQs)

be employed to liaise with the school nurse team and education welfare workers on a project to reduce the numbers of children missing school for health reasons.

Specialist school nurses are needed to assess the whole school and community, and plan improved public health outcomes, and to do specialist work such as child protection. However, the delivery of the range of interventions can be supported by other staff. Some teams employ nursery nurses to work with children from nursery age to eight years old, covering issues such as supporting parenting, advising on eating, exercise, sleeping, headlice, hygiene and liaising on issues such as enuresis. Health care support workers (sometimes called school health technicians) are employed to do routine tasks such as the weighing and measuring of 5 and 11 year olds. Community staff nurses are often employed to deliver school based immunisations. Some teams employ children's nurses in special schools and health care support workers to work with them

Specific roles

Specialist practitioner, team leader or CPD (SCPHN), *Agenda for Change* (AfC) Level 7

- To organise the operational work of the team.
- To mentor, supervise and teach specialist community public health nurses in training.
- To supervise placements of other nurses in training.
- To ensure that the school nursing service is delivering on the Trust's/employing authorites priorities on public health and health protection.
- To supply audits and other information about the school nursing service to the children's services manager.
- To make efforts to find out the views of young people in order that the service is responding to their needs.
- To attend PCT meetings and feed back to the team.
- To attend inter-agency meetings and feed back to the team.
- To develop protocols for the skill mix team.
- To plan the immunisation programme.
- To be responsible for ensuring that all team members are up to date with training requirements.
- To do personal development plans with each team member, annually and follow through with necessary action.
- To offer clinical supervision on child protection issues each half term to each qualified nurse.
- To hold a small or specialist caseload.

Specialist practitioner (SCPHN), AfC Level 6

To organise the work of a small skill mix team within a given area.

- To hold a caseload.
- To carry out school health profiles on all schools in area not just those on own caseload.
- To plan action to improve health inequalities which show up from profiles.

- To design a service level agreement with each school.
- To give high quality health education lessons to students, working in partnership with teaching staff.
- To give high quality health advice and support to school staff.
- To carry out drop-in sessions in schools and community settings, and give high quality advice and information.
- To design packages of care for disabled children.
- To delegate work appropriately.
- To ensure that school staff nurses and community nursery nurses are carrying out the work as intended.
- To be responsible for all child protection issues on caseload, and delegate to school staff nurses if they are deemed competent.

School staff nurse, AfC Level 5

Many nurses who do this job have no training in child health so it is important that levels of competency are taken into consideration when allocating caseloads. These nurses should not have "difficult" schools until they have become experienced.

- To hold a caseload (but all problems and complications to be discussed with SCPHN).
- To assist in profiling school caseload.
- To undertake health education where competent to do so, using evaluated lesson plans and toolkits, and working in conjunction with school staff.
- Support and give advice and training on first aid to school staff.
- Undertake immunisations and talk to the class beforehand in order to achieve "informed consent".
- Support children with chronic and complex conditions such as diabetes and asthma.
- To undertake child protection work where competent (which would not be the case for the first year), on the understanding that the nurse is a "novice", and must always discuss the case and his/her input with the specialist practice nurse.
- Support children and young people to complete their personal health plans.
- Review the status of all children at school entry (by discussion with teacher and nursery nurse, and see those which have been 'flagged up').
- Follow up children persistently absent from school for sickness reasons.
- Work to deliver the outcomes from the healthy schools programme.
- Work to deliver the Trust's/employing authority's targets as advised by team leader.
- Work in inter-agency settings on projects such as "junior citizen".
- Undertake training in safeguarding, child protection, common assessment framework etc.
- Read widely, and plan time for this on work schedule.
- Apply to train as SCPHN.

Community nursery nurse, AfC Level 4

- School entrant screening and collation of forms and information.
- Health education for children in Key Stage 1 (hand washing, healthy eating, oral hygiene).
- Networking/information gathering/facilitating working with school early years' staff.
- Information sessions for parents (headlice, school food policy, purpose of school dental checks, play opportunities, signposting to services).

Frequently asked questions (FAQs)

- Individual help for parents (eg. enuresis, food fads).
- Individual help for children (under 8 years) eg. children unhappy/friendship problems, bereavement, divorce, temper tantrums at school.
- They should NOT give advice re childhood immunisations, sexual health, disabilities, first aid or clinical conditions.
- They may however attend immunisation sessions to help calm anxious children, provided they feel competent to do so.

Health care assistant, AfC Level 2

- Weighing and measuring of children, especially Year 6 for national child measurement programme.
- Packing up equipment for immunisation sessions.
- Attending immunisation sessions to look after anxious pupils.
- Cleaning equipment used in clinics and health education.
- Preparing equipment for events such as health fairs or junior citizen.
- Carrying out audits for example data collection re children's choices at lunch times.
- To deputise for clerical staff when they are off site.
- Delivering clinical care when trained and skilled to do so eg. gastrostomy feeds in special schools, suction of tracheostomy.

Admin/clerical, AfC Level 3

Because of the complexity of school nursing working across health, education and social services, an experienced administrative assistant is required who can work on his/her own initiative, pre-empt problems, plan for streams of work, use all resources to gather information etc..

- Organise dates for nurses to go into schools to do planned sessions eg. immunisations or Year 6 heights and weights.
- Managing the record filing system so that it is easy to use for all team members.
- Arranging for class lists to be available.
- Attending immunisation sessions to collate and organise the paperwork.
- Inputting child health data.
- Phoning and cancelling work if nurse is off sick.
- Making appointments eg. for enuresis clinic.
- Organising stationery.
- Organising logistics of resources/toolkits/leaflets.
- Filing and finding of records.
- Keeping record of school health records re children in and out of schools and borough/county.
- Moving records at transition stages when children move to middle or secondary school.
- Moving records when a child moves school within local education area covered by PCT or health board.
- Transferring records to "out of area" school nursing team, and keeping a record of this. Receiving records from other school nurse teams when child moves into area and recording this, and bringing to the attention of the school nurse.
- Finding out which school child attends, when forms containing out of date information are received by school nursing team.

- Sorting out post – recognising and alerting nurses to important items.
- Photocopying.
- Taking minutes at meetings.
- Finding information for school nurses eg. dental service results.
- Ordering equipment and resources.
- Organising an annual calibration of scales.
- Sorting out invoices.
- Dealing with enquiries and taking messages, but NOT giving clinical advice and information.
- Reading and recording immunisation fridge temperature re protocol.
- Ordering vaccines.
- Compiling audits and producing graphs.
- Typing letters/referrals/reports.
- Maintaining databases when asked to by nurses.
- Arranging heights and weights sessions with schools for the National Child Measurement programme.
- Arranging other sessions with schools such as hearing and vision screening where this is undertaken by the school nurse team.
- Arranging medicals in special schools; sending out invitation letters and collating responses.
- Auditing of clinics, re waiting times and referrals.

What are the public health roles within skill mix teams?

The process of community practice in homes, schools or other settings may identify information and trends which are relevant to public health. It is important for all team members to be aware of, and discuss, public health issues in order to develop a family-centred public health service.

Qualified community practitioners and health visitors need to be aware of issues and trends in order to review and develop services. Therefore, it is important that team members are aware of what information is relevant to this function and that there is regular discussion, feedback and data collection regarding public health information. This will allow trends to be identified and appropriate action to be planned.

All team members will be gathering information related to public health, that is the health of communities and the provision of local services. The use of profiles to stimulate an awareness of health needs is an integral part of community assessment and it is essential to focus the attention of planners, commissioners of services and others, to the identified health needs of the local community or school.

As family-focused public health work is developed within the health visiting and school nursing services, concern has been expressed that delegation of specific areas of work may lead to a dilution of practitioners' knowledge of local families and communities. However, a team approach could be considered advantageous in that:

- The whole team should be involved in caseload profiling (see below) and "pooling" information.
- Networks may be developed outside "traditional" health care.

Frequently asked questions (FAQs)

- There is potential for research using members of the team.
- There is potential to further develop the public health role within a multi-skilled team while ensuring individual client focused work is delegated appropriately.
- There is potential to undertake health impact assessments as a team.
- There is potential for community focused public health work.

Accurate caseload profiling involves looking at the following areas:

- Numbers of families and new births per year.
- Children's services referrals and joint assessments.
- CAF referrals/key worker roles.
- Safeguarding work and numbers of children with a child protection plan.
- Time spent on core work and delivery of the child health promotion programme.
- Postnatal depression prevention, identification and intervention work.
- Complex families.
- Numbers of vulnerable families and time spent working with them.
- Teenage conception rate and numbers of teenage parents.
- Breastfeeding initiation and duration rates.
- Infant mortality rates.
- Numbers of low birth weight babies
- Numbers of parents who smoke
- Children with special additional needs.
- Length of time a family has been on the caseload.
- Numbers of transfer in and out annually.
- Liaison work.
- Numbers of travelling/homeless families/asylum seekers.
- Time spent working with families who have English as a second language.
- Record keeping and documentation per family length of time required to write up and make referrals.
- Clinics run and clinic usage.
- Group work.
- Supervision clinical and safeguarding.
- Staff meetings
- Travel and mileage to cover caseload. area

When considering skill mix introduction a systematic review of the caseload and the work involved in meeting the caseload needs reveals useful information.

References

Adams, C (2007) CPHVA *Response to 'Facing the Future – A Review of the Role of Health Visitors'*. Unite/CPHVA, London.

Adams, A, Lugsden, E (2000) Deciding to Change your Skill Mix? *British Journal of Health Care Management,* 6 (2), 65–70.

Adams, C, Craig, I (2007) Health Visitor Cuts Affecting Vulnerable Families. *Community Practitioner,* 80, (5): 14, 16–7,

Adams, C, Craig, I (2008) A Service at Crisis Point. *Community Practitioner,* 81, (12), 34–5

Andrews, A (1995) The Road to the Courts. *Health Visitor,* 69, (1), 26.

Barlow, J, Stewart-Brown, S (2003) Why a Universal Population-approach to the Prevention of Child Abuse is Essential. *Child Abuse Review,* 12, 279–281.

Barlow, J, Kirkpatrick, S, Stewart-Brown, S and Davis, H (2005) Hard-to-Reach or Out-of-Reach? Reasons Why Women Refuse to Take Part in Early Intervention. *Children and Society,* 19, 199–210.

Bergman, R (1981) Accountability – Definitions and Dimensions. *International Nursing Review,* 28, (2), 53–59.

Bidmead, C, Cowley, S (2005) A Concept Analysis of Partnership with Clients. *Community Practitioner,* 78, (6), 203–8.

Brandon, M, Beldrson, P, Warren, C, Howe, D, Gardner, R, Dodsworth, J, Black, J (2008) *Analysing Child Deaths and Serious Injury Through Child Abuse and Neglect: What Can We Learn? A Biennial Analysis of Serious Case Reviews* 2003–2005. DCSF Research Report DCSF-RR023, London.

Booth, C (2002) Review Body for Nursing Staff, Midwives and Health Visitors and Professions Allied to Medicine. The Stationery Office.

Branson, C, Badger, B and Dobbs, F (2003) Patient Satisfaction with Skill Mix in Primary Care: a Review of the Literature. *Primary Health Care Research & Development,* 4, 329–339. doi:10.1191/1463423603pc162oa

Brocklehurst, N, Adams, C (2004) *Corporate Working in Health Visiting and Public Health Nursing Teams.* CPHVA, London.

References

Brocklehurst, N, Barlow, J, Kirkpatrick, S, Davis, H and Stewart-Brown, S (2004) The Contribution of Health Visitors to Supporting Vulnerable Children and their Families at Home. *Community Practitioner,* 77, (5), 175–179.

Brown, I (1997) Skill Mix Parent Support Initiative in Health Visiting: Evaluation Study *Health Visitor,* 70, 339–343.

Buchan, J (1999) Determining Skill Mix: Lessons from an International Review. *Human Resources for Health Development,* 3, 80–90.

Buchan, J, May, F (2000) *Determining Skill Mix in the Health Workforce: Practical Guidelines for Managers and Health Professionals.* World Health Organization, Geneva, 2000 Document. (OSD Discussion Paper 3).

Cabinet Office (2007) *Reaching Out: Think Family* Social Exclusion Task Force (June 2007). http://www.cabinetoffice.gov.uk/social_exclusion_task_force/documents/think_families/think_families.pdf

Care Quality Commission (2008) NHS Staff Survey. http://www.cqc.org.uk/usingcareservices/healthcare/nhsstaffsurveys/2008nhsstaffsurvey.cfm

Carr, S, Pearson, P (2005) Delegation: Perception and Practice in Community Nursing. *Primary Health Care Research and Development,* 6, 72–81.

Charlton, BG, Calvert, N, White, M *et al* (1994) Health Promotion Priorities for General Practice: Constructing and Using "indicative prevalences". *British Medical Journal,* 308, 1019–22.

CPHVA Professional Committee (2002) *Delegation and Professional Accountability.* Professional Briefing written by Forester, S. Amicus/CPHVA, London.

Coomber, R, Cubbin, J, Davison, N and Pearson, P (1992) *Nursing Skill Mix Review.* Newcastle Community Health. Unpublished Review.

Cowley, S (1991) A Symbolic Awareness Context Identified Through a Grounded Theory of Health Visiting. *Journal of Advanced Nursing,* 16, 648–656.

Cowley, S (2009) *Response to Marmot Review.* Unite the Union/CPHVA, London.

Cowley, S (1993) Skillmix: Value for Whom? *Health Visitor,* 66, (5), 166–168.

Cowley, S (2002) Public Health Practice in Nursing and Health Visiting. In: *Public Health Policy and Practice: a Sourcebook for Health Visitors and Community Nurses.* (Ed. Cowley, S). Baillière Tindall, London.

Cowley, S, Andrews, A (2001) A Scenario-based Analysis of Health Visiting Dilemmas. *Community Practitioner,* 74, (4) 139–142.

Cowley, S, Frost, M (2006) *The Principles of Health Visiting.* Amicus/CPHVA, London.

Cowley, S (2003) Modernising Health Visiting Education: Potential, Problems and Progress. *Community Practitioner,* 76, (1) 418–422

Cowley, S (1995) In Health Visiting, a Routine Visit is One that has Passed. *Journal of Advanced Nursing,* 22, (2), 276–284.

Cowley, S (2008) *Health Needs Assessments.* In: Cowley, S (Ed.) *Community Public Health in Policy and Practice* (2nd Edition). Baillière Tindall, Edinburgh, London.

Cowley, S, Billings J (2003) A Structured Health Needs Assessment Tool: Acceptability and Effectiveness for Health Visiting. *Journal of Advanced Nursing,* 43, (1), 82–92.

Cowley S, Caan, W. Dowling, H. Weir, H. (2007) What do health visitors do? A national survey of activities and service.. Public Health. Journal of the Royal Institute of Public Health. doi:10.1016/j.puhe.2007.03.016

Cowley, S, Adams, C (2009) *The Universal Health Visiting Service.* Unite/CPHVA website http://www.unite-cphva.org/

Cowley, S, Rudgley, D (2009) *Health Visiting Matters. Interim Report.* UKPHA, London.

Darzi, A (2008) *High Quality Care for All: NHS Next Stage Review Final Report.* Department of Health, London.

Data Protection Act 1998. The Stationery Office. http://www.opsi.gov.uk/acts/acts1998/19980029.htm

Davis, H, Spurr, P (1998) Parent Counselling: An Evaluation of a Community Child Mental Health Service. *Journal of Child Psychology and Psychiatry,* 39, (3), 365–376.

De La Cuesta, C (1993) Fringe Work: Peripheral Work in Health Visiting. *Sociology of Health and Illness,* 15, (5), 665–681.

Department for Children, Schools and Families (2007) *The Children's Plan: Building Brighter Futures.* DCSF, London. (available at www.dfes.gov.uk/publications/childrensplan)

Department for Education and Skills (2004) *Every Child Matters – Change for Children.* The Stationery Office, London.

Department for Education and Skills (2005) *Common Core of Skills and Knowledge for the Children's Workforce.* The Stationery Office, London.

Department of Health (2000) *NHS Plan.* The Stationery Office, London.

Department of Health (2001) *Health Visitor and School Nurse Practice Development Resource Packs.* The Stationery Office, London.

References

Department of Health (2003) *Tackling Health Inequalities; A Programme for Action.* Department of Health, London.

Department of Health (2003a) *The Victoria Climbié Inquiry. Report of an Inquiry by Lord Laming.* Department of Health. London.

Department of Health (2003b) *Confidentiality NHS Code of Practice.* Department of Health. London.

Department of Health (2004) *Standards for Better Health.* Department of Health, London.

Department of Health (2004a) *Choosing Health: Making Healthy Choices Easier.* The Stationery Office, London.

Department of Health (2006) *Modernising Nursing Careers: Setting the Direction.* Department of Health, London.

Department of Health (2006a). *The Regulation of the Non-medical Healthcare Professions: A Review by the Department of Health.* Department of Health, London.

Department of Health (2006b). *Good Doctors, Safer Patients: Proposals to Strengthen the System to Assure and Improve the Performance of Doctors and to Protect the Safety of Patients.* Department of Health, London.

Department of Health (2007) *Facing the Future; A Review of the Role of Health Visitors.* Department of Health. www.dh.gov.uk/cno

Department of Health (2007a) *Trust Assurance and Safety the Regulation of Health Care Professionals for the 21st Century.* Department of Health, London.

Department of Health (2007b) *Safeguarding Patients: The Government's Response to the Recommendations of the Shipman Inquiry's Fifth Report and to the Recommendations of the Ayling, Neale and Kerr/Haslam Inquiries.* The Stationery Office, London.

Department of Health (2008) *Our NHS, Our Future. NHS Next Stage Review Leading Local Change.* Department of Health, London.

Department of Health (2008a) *NHS Next Stage Review Our Vision for Primary and Community Care.* Department of Health, London.

Department of Health (2009) *NHS Constitution.* Department of Health, London.

Department of Health, Unite the Union/CPHVA (2009) Joint Statement Unite/CPHVA and DH for 'Action on Health Visiting Programme'. http://www.unite-cphva.org/docs/Action%20on%20Health%20Visiting%20final%20statement.doc

Department of Health (2009) *Transforming Community Services: Ambition, Action, Achievement Series.* Department of Health, London.

Durdle Davis (2007) CPHVA *Annual Omnibus. Confidential Questionnaire.* Durdle Davis, Hereford.

European Higher Education Area (1999) Bologna Declaration. http://www.bologna-bergen2005.no/Docs/00 Main_doc/990719BOLOGNA_DECLARATION.PDF

Freedom of Information Act (2000) The Stationery Office

Future Vision Coalition (2008) *A New Vision for Mental Health* http://www.newvisionformentalhealth.org.uk/A_new_vision_for_mental_health.pdf (Accessed September 5th 2008)

Gibbs, I, McCaughan, D, Griffiths, M (1991) Skill Mix in Nursing: A Selective Review of the Literature. *Journal of Advanced Nursing,* 16, (2), 242–9.

Gimson, S (2007) *Health Visitors: An Endangered Species.* Family and Parenting Institute.

Goodwin, S (1991) Breaking the Links Between Social Deprivation and Poor Child Health. *Health Visitor,* 64, 11, 376–80.

Griffiths, P, Jones, S, Maben, J, Murrells, T (2008) *State of the Art Metrics for Nursing: A Rapid Appraisal.* National Nursing Research Unit. King's College, London. http://www.kcl.ac.uk/content/1/c6/04/32/16/NursesinsocietyFinalreport.pdf.

Hall, D, Elliman, D (2003) *Health for All Children.* (4th Edition). Oxford University Press.

Hawkins, S, Restall, M (2006) Volunteers Across the NHS; Improving the Patient Experience and Creating a Patient Led Service. Volunteering England. http://www.volunteering.org.uk/WhatWeDo/Projects+and+initiatives/volunteeringinhealth/

Healthcare Commission National Survey of NHS Staff 2006. http://www.healthcarecommission.org.uk/nationalfindings/surveys/healtheprofessionals/surveysofnhsstaff/2006.cfm

Healthcare Commission (2007) *Criteria for Assessing Core Standards in 2007/2008 Primary Care Trusts.* http://www.healthcarecommission.org.uk/_db/_documents/PCTs_criteria_for_assessing_core_standards_2007_2008.pdf

Health and Safety Executive (1974) Health and Safety at Work etc Act 1974. http://www.hse.gov.uk/legislation/hswa.pdf

Hicks, C, Hennessy, D (2000) An Alternative Methodology for Clinical Skill Mix Review: A Pilot Case Study with a Primary Health Care Team. *Journal of Interprofessional Care,* 14, (1), 59–74.

HM Government (1998) *Data Protection Act 1998.* Office of Public Sector Information (www.dataprotection.gov.uk/)

References

HM Government (1998) *Human Rights Act 1998.* Office of Public Sector Information http://www.opsi.gov.uk/acts/acts1998/ukpga_19980042_en_1

HM Government (2004) *Children Act.* Office of Public Sector Information. http://www.opsi.gov.uk/acts/acts2004/ukpga_20040031_en_1

HM Government (2006) *Reaching Out: An Action Plan on Social Exclusion.* Cabinet Office, London.

HM Government (2006) *National Health Service Act.* Office of Public Sector Information.

HM Government (2007) *Reaching Out: Think Family.* Cabinet Office, London.

HM Government (2007a) *PSA Delivery Agreement 19: Ensure Better Care for All.* HM Treasury, HMSO, Norwich.

HM Government (2008) *Information Sharing Guidance for Practitioners and Managers.* www.everychildmatters.gov.uk/informationsharing

House of Commons Health Committee (2009) *Health Inequalities: Third Report of Session 2008–2009* (Vol 1. HC 286–1). The Stationery Office, London.

Houston, A, Cowley, S (2002) An Empowerment Approach to Needs Assessment in Health Visiting Practice. *Journal of Clinical Nursing*, 10, 140–151.

Irwin, L, Siddiqi, A, Hertzman, C (2007) *Early Child Development: A Powerful Equalizer.* Final Report for the World Health Organization's Commission on the Social Determinants of Health.

Jack, S, DiCenso A and Lohfeld, L (2005) A Theory of Maternal Engagement with Public Health Nurses and Family Visitors. *Journal of Advanced Nursing*, 49, (2), 182–190.

Kennedy, A, Rogers, A and Gately, C (2005) From Patients to Providers: Prospects for Self-Care Skills Trainers in the National Health Service. *Health and Social Care in the Community*, 13, (5), 431–440.

Kirkpatrick, S, Barlow, J, Stewart-Brown, S and Davis, H (2007) Working in Partnership: User Perceptions of Intensive Home Visiting. *Child Abuse Review*, 16, 32–46.

Lord Laming (2009) *The Protection of Children in England: A Progress Report.* (HC330). The Stationery Office, London.

Longley, M, Shaw, C and Dolan, G (2007) *Nursing: Towards 2015.* Welsh Institute for Health and Social Care. University of Glamorgan.

Luker, K, Chalmers, K (1990) Gaining Access to Clients: The Case of Health Visiting. *Journal of Advanced Nursing*, 15, 74–82.

McFarlene, J (1986) *Models for Nursing.* In: Kershaw, B (Ed). John Wiley, Chichester.

MacKenzie, M (2006) Benefit or Burden: Introducing Paraprofessional Support Staff to Health Visiting Teams: The Case of Starting Well. *Health and Social Care in the Community,* 14, (6), 523–531.

McKenna, H (1995) Skill Mix Substitution and Quality of Care: An Exploration of Assumptions from the Research Literature. *Journal of Advanced Nursing,* 21: 452–59.

McKenna, H (1998) The "Professional Cleansing" of nurses. *British Medical Journal,* 317: 7170, 1403–4.

McKnight, J (2006) Skill Mix: In Whose Best Interests? *Community Practitioner,* 79, (5), 157–160.

Morell, D (1993) *Diagnosis in General Practice: Art or Science?* Nuffield Provincial Hospital Trust, London.

Netmums.com (2007) Families Need Health Visitors. http://www.netmums.com/h/n/SUPPORT/HOME/ALL/547//

Newland, R (2007) *Record Keeping & the Law.* Unite/CPHVA, London.

Newland, R (2007a) *Record Keeping and Documentation: Principles into Practice.* Unite/CPHVA, London.

Newland, R (2008) *Professional Briefing; The New Birth Visit.* Unite/CPHVA, London.

Newland, R (2009) *Exploring the Role of the Health Visitor and the Registered Nurse in the Health Visitor Team and the Health Visitor Service.* Unite/CPHVA, London

NHS (2006) Working in Partnership Programme http://www.wipp.nhs.uk/uploads/%20tools/Drafting%20your%20PDP%20as%20an%20.pdf

NHS Business Services Authority (2009) Caldicott Policy. NHS Business Services Authority.

NHS Executive (1992) *The Nursing Skill Mix in the District Nursing Service.* Value for Money Unit, HMSO.

Nursing & Midwifery Council (2004) *Standards of Proficiency for Specialist Community Public Health Nurses Education.* NMC, London

Nursing & Midwifery Council (2004) *Standards of Proficiency for Pre-Registration Nursing Education.* NMC, London.

NMC Record Keeping Guidance for Nurses and Midwives (2009) http://www.nmc-uk.org/aDisplayDocument.aspx?DocumentID=6269

References

Nursing & Midwifery Council (2007) NMC *Issues, New Advice for Delegation to Non-regulated Health Care Staff.* NMC Press Release August 2007. http://www.nmc-uk.org/aArticle.aspx?ArticleID=2582&Keyword=non%20and%20regulated%20and%20healthealthcare assistantre%20and%20staff%20and%20%20delegation (Accessed 26th August 2007)

Nursing & Midwifery Council (2008) *Advice on Delegation for Registered Nurses and Midwives* http://www.nmc-uk.org/aDisplayDocument.aspx?DocumentID=4184

Nursing & Midwifery Council (2008) *The Code. Standards of Conduct, Performance and Ethics for Nurses and Midwives.* (NMC, April 7th 2008).

Nursing & Midwifery Council (2009) *Record Keeping: Notes and FAQ. Personal and Professional Knowledge and Skills* 33. *What is the NMC's View on Students and Health Care Support Workers (HCSW) in Relation to Record Keeping?* http://www.nmc-uk.org/aArticle.aspx?ArticleID=3806

Olds, DL, Robinson, J, O'Brien, R, Luckey, DW, Pettitt, LM et al (2002) Home Visiting by Paraprofessionals and by Nurses: A Randomized, Controlled Trial. *Pediatrics,* 110, 486–96.

Olds, DL (2006) The Nurse-Family Partnership: An Evidence Based Preventive Intervention. *Infant Mental Health Journal,* 27, 5–25.

Rose, G (1993) *The Strategy of Preventative Medicine.* Oxford University Press, Oxford.

Royal College of Nursing/The Chartered Society of Physiotherapy/Royal College of Speech and Language Therapists/British Dietetic Association (2006) *Supervision, Accountability and Delegation of Activities to Support Workers. A Guide for Registered Practitioners and Support Workers.* http://www.rcn.org.uk/_data/assets/pdf_file/0006/78720/003093.pdf (Accessed September 11th 2009)

Russell, S (2008) *Left Fending for Ourselves: A Report on the Health Visitor Service as Experienced by Mums.* Netmums. http://www.netmums.com/files/FendingforOurselves_withappendix.pdf

Skills for Care and Development and Skills for Health. http://www.skillsforcare.org.uk/home/home.asp (Accessed September 2009)

Suppiah, C (1994) Working in Partnership with Community Mothers. *Health Visitor,* 67, (2) 51–53.

UKCC (1999) *Fitness for Practice.* UKCC, London.

Unite/CPHVA (2006) *Competency Framework and Best Practice Guidelines For Community Nursery Nurses.* (October 2006)

Unite/CPHVA (2007) *Cornish School Nurse Situation "Deteriorating".* Press Release Jan. 2007, Unite/CPHVA, London.

Unite/CPHVA (2007) Fact Sheet *Determining Optimum Case Load Size.* Unite/CPHVA, London.

Unite/CPHVA (2007) Professional Briefing. *Guidelines for Managing Vacant Caseloads.* Unite/CPHVA, London.

Unite/CPHVA (2007) *Managing Safely Fact Sheet. The Essentials You Need To Know.* Unite/CPHVA, London.

Unite/CPHVA (2007) Version 2. *Community Nursery Nurses. A Voluntary Code of Professional Conduct.* Unite/CPHVA, London.

Unite/CPHVA (2007) Version 2 *Community Nursery Nurses. Professional Guidelines.* Unite/CPHVA, London.

Unite/CPHVA (2007) *Recommended Induction Programme For Community Nursery Nurses.* Unite/CPHVA, London.

Unite/CPHVA (2007) *Community Practitioners' and Health Visitors' Association Response to Facing the Future: A Review of the Role of Health Visitors October 2007.* Unite/CPHVA, London.

Unite/CPHVA Health Visitors' Forum (2008) *The Distinctive Contribution of Health Visiting to Public Health and Wellbeing: A Guide for Commissioners.* Unite/CPHVA, London.

Unite/CPHVA (2008) *Every 27 Hours a Health Visitor Job is Being Lost.* Press Release April, 2008.

Unite/CPHVA (2009) *The "Final Wake-Up" as New Figures Show a Health Visitor Job is "Lost" Every 30 Hours.* Press Release March, 2009.

Unite/CPHVA (2009) *London Health Visiting Crisis Exposed by Unite.* Press Release August, 2009.

Wanless, D (2004) *Securing Good Health for the Whole Population.* HM Treasury, London.

Warner, M, Gould, E and Picek, A (1998) *Healthcare Futures 2010.* Welsh Institute for Health and Social Care, University of Glamorgan,

Watson, R (2002) Clinical Competence: Starship Enterprise or Straitjacket? *Nurse Education Today,* (6): 476–480.

Working in Partnership Programme Health Care Assistant Toolkit. http://www.rcn.org.uk/development/hca_toolkit

Wright, S (1998) Skill Mix in Health Visiting. *Journal of Community Nursing*

Relevant Unite/ CPHVA publications for further reading

Available for purchase from the Unite/CPHVA bookshop at: http://www.cairnsbookshop.co.uk/

1. Record Keeping and Documentation: Principles into Practice, Newland, R. Published 2007 Members £15, Non members – £17.50
2. The Principles of Health Visiting: Opening the Door to Public Health Practice in the 21st Century Published 2006 Members £10, Non members – £15

Free for Unite/CPHVA members from http://www.unite-cphva.org/

1. Exploring the Role of the Health Visitor and the Registered Nurse in the Health Visitor Team and the Health Visitor Service (2009)
2. The New Birth Visit (2008)
3. Guidelines for Vacant Caseloads (2006)
4. Competency Framework for Nursery Nurses (2006)
5. Community Nursery Nurse Induction Programme (2007)
6. Community Nursery Nurse (CNN) Handbook (2009)
7. What is the Unique Contribution of the Health Visitor to the Health and Wellbeing of Pre-school Children and their Families? (2009)
8. The Distinctive Contribution of Health Visiting to Public Health and Wellbeing: a Guide for Commissioners (2008)
9. CPHVA Response to Facing the Future: A Review of Health Visiting (2007)
10. Record Keeping & the Law (2009)
11. What is the Unique Contribution of the School Nurse (2009)
12. The Universal Health Visiting Service (2009)

Glossary

Competence – a bringing together of general attributes – knowledge, skills and attitudes. Skill without knowledge, understanding and the appropriate attitude does not equate with competent practice. Thus, competence is 'the skills and ability to practise safely and effectively without the need for direct supervision' (UKCC, 1999; Watson 2002).

Delegation – the transfer to a competent individual, the authority to perform a specific task in a specified situation that can be carried out in the absence of that nurse or midwife and without direct supervision.

People/person – the terms people/person has been used to represent all recipients of care including children and young people and those in acute and community settings.

Non-registered health care staff – a group of care providers that are neither registered or licensed by a regulatory body and have no legally defined scope of practice. Includes titles such as Health care assistant, Support Workers, Associate Practitioners, Assistant Practitioners, and Nursing Assistants.

Accountability – the principle that individuals, organisations and the community are responsible for their actions and may be required to explain them to others.

Responsibility – a form of trustworthiness; the trait of being answerable to someone for something or being responsible for one's conduct

Fitness to practise – fitness is a nurse or midwifes suitability to be on the register without restrictions. The NMC deals with allegations that a nurse or midwifes fitness to practise is impaired.